Molecular Imaging and Precision Medicine, Part II

Editor

RATHAN M. SUBRAMANIAM

PET CLINICS

www.pet.theclinics.com

Consulting Editor
ABASS ALAVI

October 2017 • Volume 12 • Number 4

ELSEVIER

1600 John F. Kennedy Boulevard ● Suite 1800 ● Philadelphia, Pennsylvania, 19103-2899

http://www.pet.theclinics.com

PET CLINICS Volume 12, Number 4
October 2017 ISSN 1556-8598, ISBN-13: 978-0-323-54680-5

Editor: John Vassallo (j.vassallo@elsevier.com)
Developmental Editor: Casey Potter

PET Clinics (ISSN 1556-8598) is published quarterly by Elsevier Inc., 360 Park Avenue South, New York, NY 10010-1710. Months of issue are January, April, July, and October. Periodicals postage paid at New York, NY, and additional mailing offices. Subscription prices per year are $232.00 (US individuals), $381.00 (US institutions), $100.00 (US students), $263.00 (Canadian individuals), $428.00 (Canadian institutions), $140.00 (Canadian students), $268.00 (foreign individuals), $428.00 (foreign institutions), and $140.00 (foreign students). To receive student and resident rate, orders must be accompanied by name of affiliated institution, date of term, and the signature of program/residency coordinator on institution letterhead. Orders will be billed at individual rate until proof of status is received. Foreign air speed delivery is included in all Clinics subscription prices. All prices are subject to change without notice. POSTMASTER: Send address changes to PET Clinics, Elsevier Health Sciences Division, Subscription Customer Service, 3251 Riverport Lane, Maryland Heights, MO 63043. **Customer Service: 1-800-654-2452 (U.S. and Canada); 314-447-8871 (outside U.S. and Canada). Fax: 314-447-8029. E-mail: journalscustomerservice-usa@elsevier.com (for print support); journalsonlinesupport-usa@elsevier.com (for online support).**

Reprints. For copies of 100 or more of articles in this publication, please contact the Commercial Reprints Department, Elsevier Inc., 360 Park Avenue South, New York, NY 10010-1710. Tel.: 212-633-3874; Fax: 212-633-3820; E-mail: reprints@elsevier.com.

PET Clinics is covered in MEDLINE/PubMed (Index Medicus).

Contributors

CONSULTING EDITOR

ABASS ALAVI, MD, MD (Hon), PhD (Hon), DSc (Hon)
Professor of Radiology and Neurology, Division of Nuclear Medicine, Department of Radiology, Hospital of the University of Pennsylvania, Perelman School of Medicine at the University of Pennsylvania, Philadelphia, Pennsylvania, USA

EDITOR

RATHAN M. SUBRAMANIAM, MD, PhD, MPH
Departments of Radiology, Clinical Sciences, Biomedical Engineering, and Nuclear Medicine, Advanced Imaging Research Center, Harold C. Simmons Comprehensive Cancer Center, The University of Texas Southwestern Medical Center, Dallas, Texas, USA; The Russell H. Morgan Department of Radiology and Radiological Sciences, The Johns Hopkins University School of Medicine, Baltimore, Maryland, USA

AUTHORS

ELIZABETH H. DIBBLE, MD
Department of Diagnostic Imaging, The Warren Alpert Medical School of Brown University, Rhode Island Hospital, Providence, Rhode Island, USA

LAURA EISENMENGER, MD
Department of Radiology and Biomedical Imaging, University of California San Francisco, San Francisco, California, USA

REEMA GOEL, MD
Department of Radiology, The University of Texas Southwestern Medical Center, Dallas, Texas, USA

THOMAS A. HOPE, MD
Department of Radiology and Biomedical Imaging, University of California San Francisco, Department of Radiology, San Francisco VA Health Care System, San Francisco, California, USA

EUGENE HUO, MD
Department of Radiology and Biomedical Imaging, University of California San Francisco, San Francisco, California, USA

ASHA KANDATHIL, MD
Department of Radiology, The University of Texas Southwestern Medical Center, Dallas, Texas, USA

CHUN K. KIM, MD
Division of Nuclear Medicine and Molecular
Imaging, Department of Radiology, Brigham
and Women's Hospital, Harvard Medical
School, Boston, Massachusetts, USA

CHARLES MARCUS, MD
The Russell H. Morgan Department of
Radiology and Radiological Sciences,
The Johns Hopkins University School of
Medicine, Nuclear Medicine Resident,
Department of Nuclear Medicine, Johns
Hopkins Medical Institutions, Baltimore,
Maryland, USA

ESTHER MENA, MD
Molecular Imaging Program, National Cancer
Institute, National Institutes of Health,
Bethesda, Maryland, USA

DANIELLA F. PINHO, MD
Department of Radiology, The University of
Texas Southwestern Medical Center, Dallas,
Texas, USA

YASEMIN SANLI, MD
Department of Nuclear Medicine, Medical
Faculty of Istanbul, Istanbul University,
Istanbul, Turkey; Department of Radiology,
The University of Texas Southwestern
Medical Center, Dallas, Texas, USA

**RATHAN M. SUBRAMANIAM, MD, PhD,
MPH**
Departments of Radiology, Clinical Sciences,
Biomedical Engineering, and Nuclear
Medicine, Advanced Imaging Research
Center, Harold C. Simmons Comprehensive
Cancer Center, The University of Texas
Southwestern Medical Center, Dallas, Texas,
USA; The Russell H. Morgan Department of
Radiology and Radiological Sciences, The
Johns Hopkins University School of Medicine,
Baltimore, Maryland, USA

JASON W. WACHSMANN, MD
Department of Radiology, The University of
Texas Southwestern Medical Center, Dallas,
Texas, USA

DAVID M. WILSON, MD
Department of Radiology and Biomedical
Imaging, University of California San Francisco,
San Francisco, California, USA

EBRU YILMAZ, MD
Department of Nuclear Medicine, Medical
Faculty of Istanbul, Istanbul University,
Istanbul, Turkey

DON C. YOO, MD
Associate Professor of Diagnostic Imaging
(Clinical), Department of Diagnostic Imaging,
The Warren Alpert Medical School of Brown
University, Rhode Island Hospital, Providence,
Rhode Island, USA

KATHERINE A. ZUKOTYNSKI, MD, FRCPC
Division of Nuclear Medicine and Molecular
Imaging, Departments of Medicine and
Radiology, McMaster University, Hamilton,
Ontario, Canada

Contents

Esophageal cancer commonly has a poor prognosis, which requires an accurate diagnosis and early treatment to improve outcome. Other modalities for staging, such as endoscopic ultrasound imaging and computed tomography (CT) scans, have a role in diagnosis and staging. However, PET with fluorine-18 fluoro-2-deoxy-D-glucose/CT (FDG PET/CT) scanning allows for improved detection of distant metastatic disease and can help to prevent unnecessary interventions that would increase morbidity. FDG PET/CT scanning is valuable in the neoadjuvant chemotherapy assessment and predicting survival outcomes subsequent to surgery. FDG PET/CT scanning detects recurrent disease and metastases in follow-up.

Gynecologic cancer is a heterogeneous group of diseases both functionally and morphologically. Today, PET coupled with computed tomography (PET/CT) or PET/MR imaging plays a central role in the precision medicine algorithm of patients with gynecologic malignancy. In particular, PET/CT and PET/MR imaging are molecular imaging techniques that not only are useful tools for initial staging and restaging but also provide anatomofunctional insight and can serve as predictive and prognostic biomarkers of response in patients with gynecologic malignancy.

^{18}F-FDG PET/CT has been described as an accurate tool for initial diagnosis of pancreatic adenocarcinoma. It differentiates benign from malignant causes; detects local and, especially, distant spread of disease; and is a very good predictor of patient prognosis. Pancreatic neuroendocrine tumors are rare tumors that originate from the islet cells of the pancreas. Currently, ^{68}Ga-DOTA-labeled somatostatin analogues are considered the best modality for detection of well-differentiated neuroendocrine tumors. ^{18}F-FDG PET/CT has a role in patients with poorly differentiated tumors. Recent studies have demonstrated improved survival in patients with metastatic neuroendocrine tumors treated with radiolabeled somatostatin analogues.

Fluorine-18 fluorodeoxyglucose (^{18}F-FDG) PET–computed tomography (CT) plays a significant role in diagnosis, staging, therapy selection, and therapy assessment of multiple pediatric malignancies and facilitating precision medicine delivery in pediatric patients. In patients with Hodgkin lymphoma, interim fludeoxyglucose ^{18}F-FDG PET/CT is highly sensitive and specific for predicting survival, and multiple trials with FDG PET/CT–based adaptive therapies are currently ongoing. It is superior to iodine-131 metaiodobenzylguanidine (^{131}I-MIBG) scintigraphy and bone scintigraphy for detecting metastases in neuroblastoma patients and sarcoma patients. It may predict histologic differentiation and neoadjuvant therapy assessment in Wilms tumor.

Gastric cancer is a disease with low survival rates and high morbidity, requiring accurate and prompt diagnosis and treatment. Although limited in the evaluation of the primary tumor as such, the metabolic information of primary tumors in an ^{18}F-FDG PET/CT study can assist in surgical and treatment planning and differentiating gastric cancers. It detects nodal disease with good specificity and positive predictive value, thus enabling appropriate therapy for individual patients. It provides valuable information about distant metastases, altering therapy decisions. It has reasonably good performance in detecting recurrent disease and in the follow-up of patients.

Recent advances in genomic profiling and sequencing of melanoma have provided new insights into the development of the basis for molecular biology to more accurately subgroup patients with melanoma. The development of novel mutation-targeted and immunomodulation therapy as a major component of precision oncology has revolutionized the management and outcome of patients with metastatic melanoma. PET imaging plays an important role in noninvasively assessing the tumor biological behavior, to guide individualized treatment and assess response to therapy. This review summarizes the recent genomic discoveries in melanoma in the era of targeted therapy and their implications for functional PET imaging.

PET/computed tomography (CT) can evaluate the metabolic and anatomic involvement of a variety of inflammatory, infectious, and malignant cardiovascular disorders. PET/CT is useful in evaluating coronary vasculature, hibernating myocardium, cardiac sarcoidosis, cardiac amyloidosis, cerebrovascular disease, acute aortic syndromes, cardiac and vascular neoplasms, cardiac and vascular infections, and vasculitis. Novel targeted radiopharmaceutical agents and novel use of established techniques show promise in diagnosing and monitoring cardiovascular diseases.

Skeletal and soft tissue sarcomas need early and accurate diagnosis, staging, and treatment for optimal outcome. ^{18}F-FDG PET/computed tomography (CT) is indicated in staging of patients with high-grade sarcomas and acts as a surrogate marker of histopathologic grade, guiding biopsy to most aggressive portion of the tumor. Pretherapy and posttherapy ^{18}F-FDG PET/CT metabolic parameters are reliable indicators of survival in patients with sarcoma with an important role in post-treatment response assessment, enabling the treatment plan to be modified in non-responders. ^{18}F-FDG PET/CT is particularly useful in the evaluation of molecular targeted therapies, which induce metabolic change before structural change.

The Role of PET/MR Imaging in Precision Medicine

Eugene Huo, David M. Wilson, Laura Eisenmenger, and Thomas A. Hope

Fluorodeoxyglucose PET and PET/computed tomography have gained acceptance in the evaluation of disease. Nontargeted tracers have been used in the diagnosis of certain malignancies but may not be sensitive or specific enough to become standard of care. Newer targeted PET tracers have been developed that target disease-specific biomarkers and allow accurate and sensitive detection of disease. Combined with the capabilities of MR imaging to evaluate soft tissue, precision imaging with PET/MR imaging can change the diagnosis. This article discusses specific areas in which precision imaging with nontargeted and targeted diagnostic agents can change the diagnosis and treatment.

PET CLINICS

THE CLINICS ARE AVAILABLE ONLINE!
Access your subscription at:
www.theclinics.com

3. Complete the CME Test and Evaluation. Participants must achieve a score of 70% on the test. All CME Tests and Evaluations must be completed online.

CME INQUIRIES/SPECIAL NEEDS

For all CME inquiries or special needs, please contact elsevierCME@elsevier.com.

Preface

Precision Medicine and PET/ Computed Tomography: Emerging Themes for Future Clinical Practice

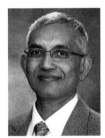

Rathan M. Subramaniam, MD, PhD, MPH
Editor

Dr R.M. Subramaniam is supported by U10 CA180870.

In this second issue of a two-part series of *PET Clinics*, which is dedicated to collate the immense value of PET/CT for implementation of precision medicine, we cover esophageal cancer, gastric cancer, and pancreatic cancer, including neuroendocrine tumors, melanoma, sarcoma, uterine and ovarian cancers, cardiovascular disorders, and PET/MR imaging. Emerging themes include nuclear medicine theragnostics, PET/MR imaging, and artificial intelligence and data analytics.

The neuroendocrine tumors paved the first wave of nuclear medicine theragnostics: diagnosis with ^{68}Ga DOTATATE PET/CT facilitating targets with expression of somatostatin receptors and peptide receptor radionucleide therapy with ^{177}Lu DOTA-TATE, a beta emitter. ^{68}Ga DOTATATE was approved by the US Food and Drug Administration (FDA) in 2016 and is now reimbursed by the US Centers for Medicare and Medicaid Services. In a recently concluded randomized controlled phase 3 trial of ^{177}Lu-DOTATATE for midgut neuroendocrine tumors, 229 patients,[1] who had well-differentiated, metastatic midgut neuroendocrine

tumors, received either ^{177}Lu-DOTATATE (116 patients) at a dose of 7.4 GBq every 8 weeks (four intravenous infusions, plus best supportive care including octreotide long-acting repeatable [LAR] administered intramuscularly at a dose of 30 mg) (^{177}Lu-DOTATATE group) or octreotide LAR alone (113 patients) administered intramuscularly at a dose of 60 mg every 4 weeks (control group). The estimated rate of progression-free survival at month 20 was 65.2% in the ^{177}Lu-DOTATATE group and 10.8% in the control group. The response rate was 18% in the ^{177}Lu-DOTATATE group versus 3% in the control group ($P<.001$). In the planned interim analysis of overall survival, 14 deaths occurred in the ^{177}Lu-DOTATATE group and 26 in the control group ($P = .004$). This is a landmark trial for the field of theragnostic nuclear medicine and molecular imaging and likely will lead to US FDA approval of ^{177}Lu-DOTATATE therapy in the future.

PET/MR imaging provides superior soft tissue characterization than PET/CT can render. PET/MR imaging with precision PET radiopharmaceuticals can provide multiparametric information about tumors for diagnosis and prognosis and in combination with theragnostic

PET Clin 12 (2017) xi–xii
http://dx.doi.org/10.1016/j.cpet.2017.07.001

radiopharmaceuticals would make an impact on patient outcomes. More efforts in organizing prospective clinical studies to demonstrate the value of PET/MR imaging, improving work flow and implementations, attenuation correction improvements to reduce biases in quantitative measurements, and advanced quantitative analytics are necessary to reap the full benefits of this emerging clinical modality.

Impact of artificial intelligence using medical imaging, including PET/CT and PET/MR imaging, will facilitate precision medicine. Medical imaging data comprise about 90% of all medical data, which provide enormous opportunities exploring artificial intelligence in tumor detection, making precision therapy decisions and prognosis. Within the next 10 to 20 years, artificial intelligence will impact the medical imaging workflow and patient management.

The future of PET/CT, PET/MR imaging, and nuclear medicine theragnostics is as bright as ever we have seen.

Rathan M. Subramaniam, MD, PhD, MPH
Department of Radiology
The University of Texas
Southwestern Medical Center
5323 Harry Hines Boulevard
Dallas, TX 75390-8896, USA

E-mail address:
rathan.subramaniam@UTsouthwestern.edu

REFERENCE

1. Strosberg J, El-Haddad G, Wolin E, et al. Phase 3 trial of 177Lu-dotatate for midgut neuroendocrine tumors. N Engl J Med 2017;376(2):125–35.

PET/Computed Tomography Scanning and Precision Medicine
Esophageal Cancer

Reema Goel, MD[a],
Rathan M. Subramaniam, MD, PhD, MPH[a,b,c,d,e],
Jason W. Wachsmann, MD[a,*]

KEYWORDS

- Esophageal cancer • Esophageal carcinoma • PET • PET/CT • FDG PET/CT

KEY POINTS

- National Comprehensive Cancer Network guidelines recommend PET with fluorine-18 fluoro-2-deoxy-D-glucose/computed tomography (FDG PET/CT) scanning at baseline staging for exclusion of distant metastatic disease to prevent unnecessary interventions.
- FDG PET/CT scanning can predict neoadjuvant chemoradiotherapy assessment and survival outcome of patients who undergo subsequent surgical resection.
- FDG PET/CT scanning is valuable in detecting recurrences and metastases in follow-up.

INTRODUCTION

Esophageal malignancy ranks sixth among cancer deaths worldwide.[1] The 2 major histologic types of esophageal cancer—adenocarcinoma (AC) and squamous cell carcinoma (SCC)—are known to differ greatly in terms of risk factors and epidemiology. In 2012 alone, an estimated 398,000 SCCs and 52,000 ACs of the esophagus were diagnosed, translating to incidence rates of 5.2 and 0.7 per 100,000, respectively.[2] However, over the past 3 decades, the rates of SCC have declined, whereas those of AC have been progressively increasing.[3] There is a significantly high concentration of AC in high-income countries in North America and Europe, with gastroesophageal reflux disease and obesity being the principal risk factors.[2] SCC remains the predominant esophageal cancer in Asia, Africa, and South America as well as among African Americans in North America. Alcohol and tobacco use are the main risk factors, with esophageal squamous dysplasia identified as the precursor lesion.[4] The incidence of esophageal carcinoma increases with age, peaking in the seventh and eighth decades of life. Men are at 3 to 4 times higher risk for AC as compared with women. However, the sex distribution is more similar for SCC. Esophageal malignancies continue to have a particularly poor prognosis because early

Disclosure Statement: None.
[a] Department of Radiology, The University of Texas Southwestern Medical Center, 5323 Harry Hines Boulevard, Dallas, TX 75390-8896, USA; [b] Department of Clinical Sciences, The University of Texas Southwestern Medical Center, 5323 Harry Hines Boulevard, Dallas, TX 75390-8896, USA; [c] Department of Biomedical Engineering, The University of Texas Southwestern Medical Center, 5323 Harry Hines Boulevard, Dallas, TX 75390-8896, USA; [d] Advanced Imaging Research Center, The University of Texas Southwestern Medical Center, 5323 Harry Hines Boulevard, Dallas, TX 75390-8896, USA; [e] Harold C. Simmons Comprehensive Cancer Center, The University of Texas Southwestern Medical Center, 5323 Harry Hines Boulevard, Dallas, TX 75390-8896, USA
* Corresponding author.
E-mail address: Jason.Wachsmann@UTSouthwestern.edu

disease typically causes no symptoms and are diagnosed later in their course.[4] More than one-half of cases (ACC or SCC or both) present with distant metastases or unresectable disease. Although the 5-year survival has been increasing over time, it remains at a dismal 18%.[5]

Owing to its poor prognosis, the development of clinically applicable biomarkers for diagnosis, therapy response, and recurrence detection has been the focus of many research studies. Although advances in molecular biology and bioinformatics have led to an improved understanding of esophageal cancer genetics, its in-depth molecular characterization remains an enigma.[6] In today's emerging era of precision medicine, a better understanding of individual variability in environment, lifestyle, and genetics may help in tailoring precise management approaches. Imaging could be a major component of such an assessment technique. This review summarizes the recent molecular advances in esophageal cancer highlighting the role of molecular and functional imaging including PET with ^{18}F-flourodeoxy glucose and computed tomography (FDG PET/CT) scanning and novel PET tracers in characterizing specific molecular mechanisms for therapy selection and its follow-up response assessment.

GENOMICS
Squamous Cell Carcinoma

Tremendous progress has been made in cancer genomics in the recent past with the advent of high-throughput techniques like next-generation sequencing. However, the full repertoire of molecular events detailing the pathogenesis of SCC remains unclear. The genetic landscape of human SCC with whole-genome, exon sequencing and array-based comparative genomic hybridization has been reported.[7,8] These studies found the highest frequency of mutation in TP53, proposing mutation of TP53 as a key factor in the development of SCC. Another common genetic polymorphism noted in SCC is SOX2 polymorphism, which is an amplified lineage-survival oncogene in SCC.[9] This transcription factor is overexpressed and amplified in a subset of squamous epithelial cells of SCC, and is associated with higher histologic grade and poor survival in SCC.[10]

Other tumor-associated genes, such as RB1, CDKN2A, PIK3CA, NOTCH1, NFE2L2, ADAM29, and FAM135B, have been implicated.[8] Notably, FAM135B is identified as a novel cancer-implicated gene as assayed for its ability to promote malignancy of SCC cells. Additionally, MIR548K, a miRNA (microRNA) encoded in the amplified 11q13.3 to 13.4 region, is characterized

as a novel oncogene, and functional assays demonstrate that MIR548 K enhances malignant phenotypes of SCC cells.

Epidermal growth factor receptor (EGFR) signaling pathways are also considered to be involved in the development of SCC. It is reported to be overexpressed in 60% to 76% of SCCs and is associated with a poor prognosis.[11,12] Genomic alterations of several important pathways, including Wnt, cell cycle, Notch, RTK–Ras, and AKT pathways are detailed in **Fig. 1**.

Adenocarcinoma

The natural history of AC is poorly understood; however, it is well-known that most of these cases arise on a background of Barrett esophagus. Barrett esophagus is a readily detectable premalignant precursor and occurs when there is metaplastic transformation of stratified squamous esophageal epithelium to the intestinal epithelium, which ultimately turns into AC.[13,14] This unique feature of AC makes it a prime candidate for the exploration of novel approaches to early diagnosis (**Fig. 2**), including a combination of genomics, transcriptomics, and microbiomics, which might lead to a personalized risk stratification approach for each patient, enabling time for early intervention.

Both Barrett esophagus and AC seem to have substantial overlap in the set of genes contributing to risk of each condition.[15,16] However, genetic risk factors contributing specifically to Barrett esophagus or esophageal AC alone might also exist. So far, genome-wide association studies have identified 4 loci within or near MHC, namely, FOXF1, GDF7, and TBX5, associated with the development of Barrett esophagus, and 4 additional loci within or near CRTC1, BARX1, FOXP1, and ALDH1A2 associated with the development of both Barrett esophagus and AC.[17,18] However, no specific marker for AC has been identified.

Both Barrett esophagus and AC are characterized by loss of heterozygosity, aneuploidy, specific genetic mutations, and clonal diversity. Epigenetic as well as DNA methylation abnormalities are also frequently seen in AC.

Somatic genomic alterations
Somatic genomic alterations in AC, including recurrent amplifications, deletions, and single nucleotide variants, have been demonstrated at the loci of a number of novel as well as established oncogenes involved with cell signaling (EGFR, ERBB2, KRAS, MET, FGFR2), the cell cycle (CCND1, CDK6 and CCNE1), and transcription factors (MYC, GATA4 and GATA6).[19–24] Aneuploidy and oncogene activation seem to be

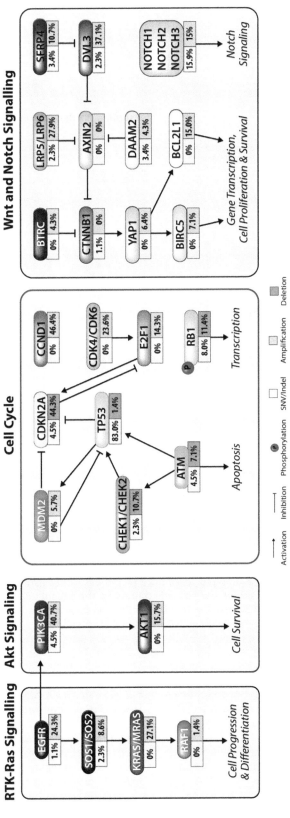

Fig. 1. Genomic alterations of important pathways in esophageal squamous cell carcinoma, including Wnt, cell cycle, Notch, RTK–Ras, and AKT pathways.

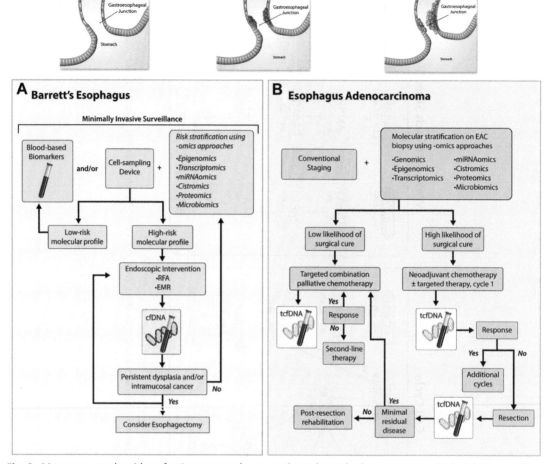

Fig. 2. Management algorithms for Barrett esophagus and esophageal adenocarcinoma (AC). (*A*) The combination of genomics, transcriptomics, and microbiomics technologies coupled with minimally invasive, unbiased sampling techniques might lead to a personalized risk stratification approach for patients with Barrett esophagus, as well as AC, enabling the detection of lesions at an earlier stage. Minimally invasive treatments of early lesions have been demonstrated to provide complete remission with minimal morbidity. The addition of cfDNA tracking might enable the assessment of completeness of this treatment. Genomic information will also identify potential targeted therapies, the response to which would be assessed using personalized tcfDNA assays. (*B*) Esophageal adenocarcinoma molecular stratification can be performed by a number of techniques, from genomics to microbiomics. From this information, a decision can be made concerning the patient's options for a surgical cure and necessity for subsequent therapies. cfDNA, cell-free DNA; EAC, esophageal adenocarcinoma; EMR, endoscopic mucosal resection; RFA, radiofrequency ablation; tcfDNA, tumor cell-free DNA.

important precursors for progression to cancer. Whole genome doubling has also been found to be a prominent feature of AC. Several studies have identified known tumor suppressors, *TP53* and *CDKN2A*, as recurrently targeted genes in AC development.[25,26]

Recent genomic studies concluded that almost one-quarter of ACs harbor at least 1 mutation in a chromatin remodeling gene. *ARID1A* and *SMARCA4*, members of the SWI/SNF (Switch/sucrose nonfermentable) complex, have been

identified as being the most frequent.[22–24] Additionally, recurrent mutations have been noted in *ELMO1* and *DOCK2*, genes feeding into the RAC1 GTPase pathway.[22]

Alterations in microRNA expression Alterations in miRNA Expression in AC have been described. There is evidence to suggest that *miR-21* and *miR-375* play a functional role in the development AC. miRNA expression profiles have been shown to be able to distinguish normal esophagus from

AC.[27,28] Differential expression of miRNAs is also associated with the progression of Barrett esophagus to AC.[29]

Epigenetic alterations occur early during progression of Barrett esophagus to AC, including hypermethylation of genes encoding ADAM (A Disintegrin And Metalloproteinase) peptidase proteins, cadherins, protocadherins, and potassium voltage-gated channels.[30] Aberrant methylation of promoter CpG islands can lead to gene silencing of a subset of genes, and is seen to occur frequently in Barrett esophagus and AC.[31,32] CpG island hypermethylation of the *CDKN2A* promoter has been reported in 3% to 77% of Barrett esophagus cases suggesting that *CDKN2A* methylation is in early event in its pathogenesis.[33] Aberrant methylation of *APC* and *CDH1* has also been evaluated in several studies.[34,35] Hypermethylated *APC* was found in 39.5% of Barrett and 92% of AC cases, and was associated with reduced survival in AC.[34]

Several studies have attempted to develop genomic or immunohistochemical signatures that might allow the segregation of patients according to prognosis.[36–40] One group of patients selected differentially expressed genes that were noted to be linked to prognosis and identified a 4-gene panel that accurately prognosticated patients. Additional prognostic markers have been identified, including *EGFR*, *MTMR9*, *WT1*, and *NEIL2*, which were also validated by immunohistochemistry.[41] These 2 datasets have been refined further to create a more clinically applicable 3 gene signature that was validated in a large, retrospective, multicenter study.[38]

STAGING AND PET/COMPUTED TOMOGRAPHY SCANNING

Staging of esophageal cancer is described using the American Joint Committee on Cancer's (AJCC) TNM system. According to the 8th edition, classifications are now termed *categories* and *subcategories*.[42,43] Criteria define the elements of categories. Esophageal anatomic cancer categories include primary tumor (T), regional lymph node (N), and distant sites of metastatic disease (M) (**Table 1**). Subcategorization of pT1 into pT1a and pT1b has been refined and improved stage I grouping. The definition of the esophagogastric junction has been revised, such that cancers with epicenters no more than 2 cm into the gastric cardia are staged as AC of the esophagus and those with more than a 2-cm involvement of the gastric cardia are staged as stomach cancers.

The National Comprehensive Cancer Network guidelines outline the detailed workup for esophageal cancer evaluation (**Box 1**). Initial staging is performed with a combination of several modalities including CT scanning of the chest, abdomen, and pelvis (if clinically indicated) using intravenous contrast to evaluate for any obvious lymphadenopathy/distant metastases.[44] Hybrid FDG PET/CT scanning is preferred, if there is no evidence of distant metastatic disease.[44] This is important in avoiding unnecessary or ineffective surgical intervention in cases with occult metastases. Distant sites of metastatic disease in esophageal cancer depend on tumor histology; SCC tends to spread within the thorax, whereas AC tends to spread within the abdomen and can involve the liver and peritoneum. Axial and proximal appendicular skeleton and adrenal glands can also be affected.[45]

In the absence of evidence of metastatic disease, locoregional staging with endoscopic ultrasound (EUS) imaging is performed, which allows for better assessment of tumor invasion and regional lymph node involvement. Fine-needle aspiration of any suspicious lymph nodes during the procedure is an added advantage of this technique. It should be noted that, although EUS is the most accurate modality for establishing the T stage of a lesion, none of the imaging modalities discussed previously are adequate for this purpose in early lesions and occasionally overestimate their depth. For that reason, endoscopic mucosal resection should be the first step for evaluation of subtle or flat lesions.[46] It allows for more accurate staging for early stage cancer.[46]

As discussed, EUS is superior to FDG PET/CT scanning for accurate staging of primary tumor and locoregional node involvement in esophageal cancer[47] (**Figs. 3** and **4**). Among primary tumors, 68% to 100% show FDG uptake, whereas early stage T1 and T2 tumors tend to have minimal or no FDG uptake likely secondary to lower degree of cellular proliferation in these smaller tumors.[48] FDG PET/CT scanning has low sensitivity of 55%, but a moderate specificity of 76% in detecting locoregional lymph node metastases.[49] Significant FDG uptake in the primary tumor often obscures increased uptake in more proximal locoregional nodes and leads to lower sensitivity.[49]

The main role of FDG PET/CT scanning in initial staging of esophageal cancer lies in its superior ability for detection of stage IV disease[50] (**Fig. 5**). The Society for Thoracic Surgeons guidelines emphasized the value of FDG PET/CT scanning owing to its higher sensitivity and specificity over other imaging modalities for the detection of distant metastases.[51] Another systematic review of nonrandomized studies reported pooled estimates for the sensitivity and specificity of FDG-PET

Table 1
Cancer staging categories for cancer of the esophagus and esophagogastric junction

Category	Criteria
T category	
TX	Tumor cannot be assessed
T0	No evidence of primary tumor
Tis	High-grade dysplasia, defined as malignant cells confined by the basement membrane
T1	Tumor invades the lamina propria, muscularis mucosae, or submucosa
T1a[a]	Tumor invades the lamina propria or muscularis mucosae
T1b[a]	Tumor invades the submucosa
T2	Tumor invades the muscularis propria
T3	Tumor invades the adventitia
T4	Tumor invades adjacent structures
T4a[a]	Tumor invades the pleura, pericardium, azygos vein, diaphragm, or peritoneum
T4b[a]	Tumor invades other adjacent structures, such as the aorta, vertebral body, or trachea
N category	
NX	Regional lymph nodes cannot be assessed
N0	No regional lymph node metastasis
N1	Metastasis in 1–2 regional lymph nodes
N2	Metastasis in 3–6 regional lymph nodes
N3	Metastasis in $\geq$7 regional lymph nodes
M category	
M0	No distant metastasis
M1	Distant metastasis
Adenocarcinoma G category	
GX	Differentiation cannot be assessed
G1	Well differentiated, with >95% of the tumor composed of well-formed glands
G2	Moderately differentiated, with 50%–95% of the tumor showing gland formation
G3[b]	Poorly differentiated, with tumors composed of nest and sheets of cells with <50% of the tumor demonstrating glandular formation
Squamous cell carcinoma G category	
GX	Differentiation cannot be assessed
G1	Well-differentiated, with prominent keratinization with pearl formation and a minor component of nonkeratinizing basallike cells, tumor cells arranged in sheets, and mitotic counts low
G2	Moderately differentiated, with variable histologic features ranging from parakeratotic to poorly keratinizing lesions and pearl formation generally absent
G3[c]	Poorly differentiated, consisting predominantly of basallike cells forming large and small nests with frequent central necrosis and with the nests consisting of sheets or pavementlike arrangements of tumor cells that are occasionally punctuated by small numbers of parakeratotic or keratinizing cells
Squamous cell carcinoma L category[d]	
LX	Location unknown
Upper	Cervical esophagus to the lower border of the azygos vein
Middle	Lower border of the azygos vein to the lower border of the inferior pulmonary vein
Lower	Lower border of the inferior pulmonary vein to the stomach, including the esophagogastric junction

[a] Subcategories.
[b] If further testing of "undifferentiated" cancers reveals a glandular component, categorize as adenocarcinoma G3.
[c] If further testing of "undifferentiated" cancers reveals a squamous cell component or if after further testing they remain undifferentiated, categorize as squamous cell carcinoma G3.
[d] Location is defined by epicenter of esophageal tumor.

scanning for stage IV disease at 67% and 97%, respectively.[52] Subsequently, the American College of Surgeons Oncology Group reported sensitivity and specificity of FDG-PET/CT scans to be 79% and 95%, respectively. This study was a multicenter prospective trial that evaluated the role of FDG PET/CT scans in detecting M1b disease among patients with biopsy-proven carcinoma of the esophagus who previously underwent CT imaging and did not have evidence of distant disease.[53] FDG PET/CT scanning has been shown to provide improved staging information and change in management in about one-third of patients, compared with EUS and CT imaging.[54] In another retrospective evaluation of 200 patients, FDG PET/CT scanning provided additional information in 37 patients (18.5%) and directly altered management in 34 (17%).[55] They also investigated the impact of tumor histology on the standardized uptake value (SUV) and found median maximum SUV (SUV_{max}) for AC to be significantly lower than that for SCC. In AC alone, the addition of FDG PET/CT imaging to standard staging procedures led to changes in multidisciplinary team recommendations in 38.2% of patients, improving patient selection for radical treatment.[56] In more recent studies, the percentage change in pretherapeutic stage by FDG PET/CT evaluation has mostly decreased to below 20%, which likely corresponds with the increasing quality of the other staging techniques, especially multislice CT scanning.[57–62]

PET with 3-deoxy-3-^{18}F-fluorothymidine/CT (FLT PET/CT) scanning has also been evaluated for esophageal cancer staging.[63] Because FLT has higher uptake in proliferating tumors and

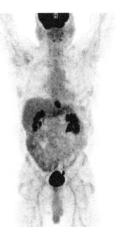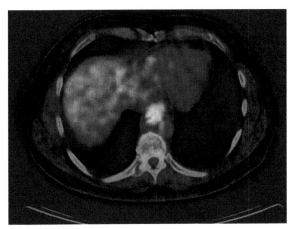

Fig. 3. A 71-year-old man diagnosed with gastroesophageal (GE) junction adenocarcinoma, moderately differentiated, underwent PET with fluorine-18 fluoro-2-deoxy-D-glucose/computed tomography (FDG PET/CT) for initial staging. It showed FDG-avid esophageal thickening at the GE junction in the maximum intensity projection image and fused PET/CT axial images without evidence of FDG-avid metastatic disease, clinically stage T3N0M0.

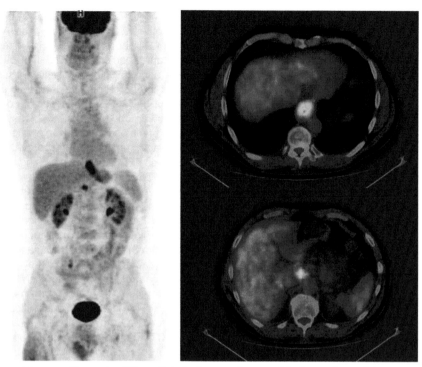

Fig. 4. A 57-year-old man with poorly differentiated adenocarcinoma with signet ring cell features of the distal esophagus with extension to the gastric cardia. Staging PET with fluorine-18 fluoro-2-deoxy-D-glucose/computed tomography (FDG PET/CT) showed intensely FDG-avid esophageal thickening involving the distal 4-cm esophagus with extension to the gastroesophageal junction and gastric cardia, as well as enlarged hypermetabolic upper abdominal node in celiac axis as seen on maximum intensity projection and fused PET/CT axial images. Subsequent esophagogastroduodenoscopy/endoscopic ultrasound imaging confirmed these findings (stage T3N2 M0).

more accurate identification of malignant tissues over benign, as shown in both in vitro and in vivo studies, it seems to have significant advantages over FDG.[64] Han and colleagues[63] compared the abilities of FLT and FDG PET/CT scanning in the detection of regional lymph node metastasis in 22 patients with SCC and found that, although FLT uptake in regional lymph nodes of esophageal carcinoma was significantly lower compared with FDG uptake, it had fewer false-positive findings and higher specificity compared with FDG PET/CT scanning. Additional work is needed to evaluate the usefulness of FLT in esophageal cancer staging, and FDG remains the current tracer of choice.

PRETHERAPY PET WITH FLUORINE-18 FLUORO-2-DEOXY-D-GLUCOSE/COMPUTED TOMOGRAPHY SCANNING AND PROGNOSIS

FDG PET/CT imaging parameters can provide valuable prognostic information before treatment. The underlying thought is that the quantity of FDG activity in the tumor correlates with viable tumor cell number and metabolism, hence with prognosis. The most commonly used (semi-)quantification parameter in clinical use is the SUV of the primary tumor.

Correlation between higher SUV (SUV_{max}), worse overall and disease-free survival has been reported in several studies.[65–70] Omloo and colleagues[71] reported that 12 of 15 studies included in their analysis showed that pretreatment SUV is a predictor for survival in univariate analysis.[72] However, only 2 of these studies showed this difference in multivariate analysis. Although pretreatment SUV may be prognostic, variable SUV_{max} thresholds have been reported as being significant. For example, significant difference in survival was shown by Rizk and colleagues,[65] who used an SUV_{max} threshold of 4.5, whereas Cerfolio and colleagues[66] suggested 6.6 as an ideal threshold.

In another study, a significant correlation was found between FDG uptake and glucose transporter 1 (GLUT-1) expression. Low GLUT-1 expression and low FDG uptake in tumors were found to have a better prognosis, showing a 100% survival at 2 years.[73] Multivariate analysis was, however, not performed. Another study investigated the role of various biological parameters

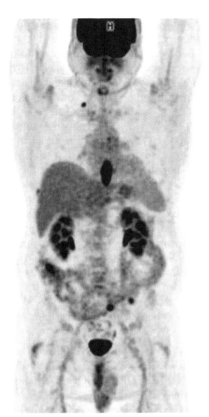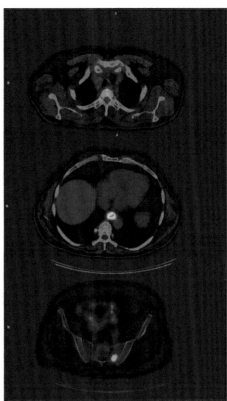

Fig. 5. A 58-year-old man with poorly differentiated adenocarcinoma of the distal esophagus was evaluated with PET with fluorine-18 fluoro-2-deoxy-D-glucose/computed tomography (FDG PET/CT). Fused FDG PET/CT images from the staging FDG PET/CT demonstrated FDG-avid distal esophageal thickening, an FDG-avid 8-mm level 2R mediastinal lymph node, and FDG-avid lytic lesion in the left sacrum (stage T3N1M0-M1).

involved in FDG uptake in esophageal AC including vascular markers such as vascular endothelial growth factor (VEGF), CD-31, GLUT-1, hexokinases (HK) isoforms I and II, Ki67, caspase-3, and CD68. The investigators found no association between FDG uptake and these markers with the exception of GLUT-1 and tumor size, for which a significant correlation was found.[69] Few studies have shown a prognostic value for VEGF assessment in esophageal SCC. However, in ACs VEGF expression patterns failed to provide any prognostic information.[74]

In another recent investigation, Schreurs and colleagues[75] suggested an SUV_{max} threshold of 3.67, which predicted a significantly lower disease-free survival and distant recurrence-free survival in 47 patients undergoing esophagectomy, as a curative intent. High HK-II expression was correlated with reduced SUV_{max} values and was significantly higher in AC compared with SCC. Preoperative high FDG uptake in primary tumors, including AC, was also noted to be associated with nodal metastases in this study. Several studies have previously reported preoperative

FDG uptake as an independent predictor of nodal metastases in SCC, but not in AC.[76,77] However, this group found no positive correlation between SUV_{max} and GLUT-1, HK-1, hypoxia inducible factor-1a, VEGF-C, p53, and Ki-67 expression.

Quantification by SUV_{max} does not account for the significant heterogeneity of FDG uptake or account for the fact that many tumors have both malignant and nonmalignant components. Spatial FDG PET features such as tumor volume, its shape, and textural features have been suggested to provide more information than SUV_{max}.[78–80] The volume of tumor with increased glycolytic activity above a specified SUV threshold also known as metabolic tumor volume (MTV) is being evaluated increasingly by investigators as a marker for prognosis in several malignancies. However, it is difficult to compare studies and evaluate the benefit of MTV owing to lack of standard threshold values. Use of MTV was first reported in 2011 in 151 patients with SCC.[81] Although the SUV_{max} and MTV were each significant predictors of survival in univariate analysis, only MTV was shown to be significant in multivariate analysis, along with T and

M stage. Similar results were obtained in another recent investigation by Malik and colleagues.[82] They concluded that MTV has more prognostic importance than SUV_{max} and provides valuable prognostic information in esophageal and junctional cancer, along with EUS T and N stage. Another FDG PET/CT parameter is total lesion glycolysis (TLG), which is MTV multiplied by the mean SUV (SUV_{mean}). Data on the use of TLG in esophageal cancer is limited. One recent study has, however, suggested that TLG may be a useful prognostic factor.[83]

RESPONSE EVALUATION

Patients who respond to neoadjuvant chemoradiation therapy (CRT) have a survival benefit and lower recurrence rates, regardless of whether they underwent resection, whereas patients who did not respond to CRT had poor prognoses, although surgery improved survival in these patients.[84–87] Identification of nonresponders early during treatment can help to appropriately select patients for surgery, thus avoiding the toxic side effects of therapy.[88,89]

Several imaging techniques used to evaluate treatment response after neoadjuvant therapy include CT, EUS, and FDG PET/CT studies. One advantage of clinical response evaluation using EUS and CT imaging is the ease of use during and after therapy and not just after resection.[90,91] However, CT scanning has a relatively poor sensitivity (33%–55%) and specificity (50%–71%) in esophageal cancer response evaluation.[92] This lack is related primarily to infiltrative growth pattern of these tumors, which makes accurate CT measurements challenging. Assessing treatment response can become more difficult after CRT compared with after chemotherapy, because therapy-induced changes such as inflammation, edema, and scarring are significantly higher.[93] In addition, many novel cancer therapies are cytostatic instead of cytocidal, and a reasonable tumor response may occur without a significant reduction in tumor size.[94] Functional imaging by FDG PET scanning provides information on the metabolic activity of tumor cells and has become a powerful treatment response evaluation tool in the recent past. In 1 large metaanalysis, FDG PET/CT scanning after CRT in patients with esophageal cancer, sensitivities and specificities ranged from 71% to 100% and 55% to 100%, respectively.[92] PET Response Criteria in Solid Tumors (PERCIST) determined that changes in peak SUV, corrected for lean body mass, was useful to evaluate tumor response.[92] PERCIST criteria have also been shown to be independent predictor

of survival in those with advanced esophageal cancer.[95]

Two ways have been identified to predict complete histopathologic response (pCR) by functional imaging: retrospectively defining cutoff values (with reported accuracies of 75%) as well as interpreting a posttherapy FDG-negative tumors as a pCR.[96–101] However, residual tumor in FDG-negative tumors is seen in a high percentage of patients demonstrating that a posttherapeutic FDG-negative tumor may not be synonymous with a pCR.[99] In contrast, increased FDG uptake can be seen after radiation therapy owing to direct esophageal injury and subsequent inflammation, and can be mistaken for residual tumor.[101] Because radiation esophagitis usually begins about 2 weeks after the initiation of therapy, and is more common with higher radiation doses, the assessment of response within the first 2 weeks of radiation treatment might prove to be more accurate and less prone to false-positive findings.[102]

PET WITH FLUORINE-18 FLUORO-2-DEOXY-D-GLUCOSE/COMPUTED TOMOGRAPHY SCANNING FOR RESPONSE EVALUATION DURING TREATMENT

It has been noted that only 40% to 50% of patients show a significant response to neoadjuvant therapy.[103] Thus, to avoid treatment-related toxicity without any significant benefit, personalizing treatment based on the use of noninvasive PET parameters would be ideal. In fact, the most clinically relevant aspect of PET imaging aside from the correct prediction of a pCR is the early treatment response evaluation.[104]

In a 2001 study conducted on patients with locally advanced AC receiving cisplatin-based neoadjuvant chemotherapy, Weber and colleagues[105] reported a cutoff decrease of 35% compared with the initial SUV to be associated with clinical and histopathologic response after 2 weeks of therapy. This cutoff was used to identify nonresponding patients accurately and was validated prospectively in an independent patient cohort by Ott and colleagues.[67,106] Metabolic responders who underwent resection had significantly higher rate of either histopathologically complete or subtotal tumor regression than those who were nonresponders (53% and 5%, respectively). This cutoff also predicted a longer time for disease progression ($P = .01$) and longer overall survival ($P = .04$). In the MUNICON I trial (Metabolic response evalUatioN for Individualisation of neoadjuvant Chemotherapy in oesOphageal and oesophagogastric adeNocarcinoma), an FDG PET/CT response–based treatment modification was included after 2 weeks, wherein metabolic nonresponders discontinued chemotherapy and underwent immediate resection.[107] Metabolic response was defined by a 35% or greater reduction in metabolic activity. When compared with historical survival data, it was shown that metabolic responders did not seem to have an overall survival disadvantage compared with nonresponding patients who completed the chemotherapy regimen over 3 months (median survival, of 26 months vs 18 months, respectively). The MUNICON II trial was devised to increase response and prognosis in metabolic nonresponders with the addition of salvage neoadjuvant CRT.[107] A major histopathologic response was observed in 26% of the metabolic nonresponders who underwent CRT, even though the progression-free survival (PFS) remained significantly worse compared with that of metabolic responders (1-year PFS, 74% vs 57%; $P = .035$). The authors concluded that salvage neoadjuvant CRT led to local remissions in a select group of patients; however, systemic disease continued to influence clinical outcomes and survival. There is an ongoing CALGB 80803 phase II trial (Cancer and Leukemia Group B), with the goal of increasing the pCR by switching the type of chemotherapy in patients with no response after 6 weeks of an assigned chemotherapy regimen (FOLFOX6 vs carboplatin/paclitaxel), based on PET response assessment. This is a different approach from that used in the previous MUNICON II trial, and the results will show if the PFS can be increased with this approach.

Investigators generally combine SCC and AC with cutoffs ranging from 0% to −35% at assessment time points of 2 to 6 weeks after the initiation of therapy.[67,105,108,109] In a study similar to previously described by Weber and colleagues,[105] Wieder and colleagues[110] performed an assessment in SCC with FDG PET/CT imaging at baseline and 2 weeks after initiation of neoadjuvant CRT (as compared with the prior study where radiation was not given). Using a slightly different metabolic response definition of 30% or greater decrease in SUV value, similar results including significantly improved survival and histopathologic response in responders as compared with nonresponders (44% and 21%, respectively; $P = .0055$) was seen. Recent data suggest that FLT PET/CT imaging may allow for better differentiation between inflammation and residual tumor during neoadjuvant treatment.[111,112]

FDG PET/CT scanning has also been used in quantifying metabolic response of tumors to targeted therapy such as to EGFR inhibitor therapies in lung cancer.[113] Several prospective studies have also assessed the value of FDG-PET in predicting survival outcomes in these category of patients and suggested that FDG PET/CT evaluation accurately identified patients who benefited from tyrosine kinase inhibitors treatment and allowed earlier response evaluation than conventional methods. FLT PET/CT scanning has also been evaluated in predicting PFS and overall survival in patients receiving targeted therapies.[114] In a retrospective review of 30 patients with stage IV non–small cell lung cancer, lower early and late residual FLT tumor uptake after 1 and 6 weeks of erlotinib therapy, respectively, were found to be associated with prolonged PFS compared with patients with higher residual tumor FLT uptake.[114]

PET WITH FLUORINE-18 FLUORO-2-DEOXY-D-GLUCOSE/COMPUTED TOMOGRAPHY SCANNING FOR RESPONSE EVALUATION AFTER TREATMENT

Most of the investigations assessing the usefulness of posttreatment FDG PET/CT imaging are single-institution, retrospective studies with fairly small numbers of patients, but they collectively suggest that uptake on FDG PET/CT scanning after neoadjuvant therapy is associated with prognosis and histopathologic response[100,115] (**Figs. 5** and **6**). A recent review of 26 studies including 1544 patients with esophageal and gastroesophageal junction cancer who received neoadjuvant therapy showed a clear association between posttherapeutic SUV (maximum and mean values) and histopathologic response.[116] In fact, the hazard ratio for complete metabolic response compared with no response was 0.51 for overall survival. In another metaanalysis of 20 studies, a pooled sensitivity and specificity of FDG PET/CT scanning in the prediction of histopathologic tumor response was shown to be 67% and 68%, respectively.[117] These results suggest that a complete metabolic response may be a better predictor of prognosis than a surrogate endpoint, such as histopathologic response.

PET WITH FLUORINE-18 FLUORO-2-DEOXY-D-GLUCOSE/COMPUTED TOMOGRAPHY SCANNING FOR RECURRENCE DETECTION AND FOLLOW-UP

PET/CT scanning is often used to monitor for recurrent or metastatic disease after esophagectomy.[118,119] Local disease recurrence, which may be a subtle finding on diagnostic CT scans alone, can better be detected by PET scans and most commonly seen near the anastomotic site. Although patients who develop recurrent disease after

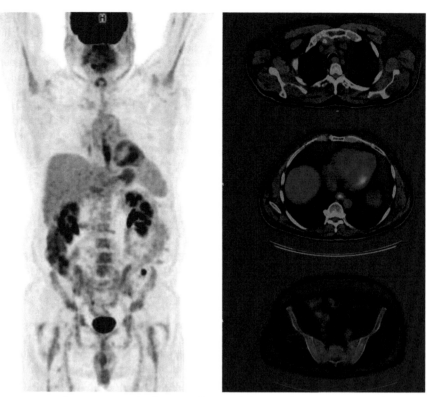

Fig. 6. On posttreatment images, 1 month after completion of chemoradiotherapy, showed treatment response with decrease in fluorine-18 fluoro-2-deoxy-ᴅ-glucose (FDG) avidity within the distal esophagus, complete resolution of 2R mediastinal lymph node, and complete resolution of metabolic activity of the left sacral lesion. Focal FDG avidity in the left colon with no computed tomography correlate seen on maximum intensity projection images was proven to be a tubular adenoma on colonoscopy.

esophagectomy are considered incurable, they may be candidates for palliative chemotherapy or radiation therapy. In such cases, FDG PET/CT has a high diagnostic accuracy; for instance, Flamen and colleagues[118] reported a sensitivity of 94%, specificity of 82%, and accuracy of 87% for detection of recurrent esophageal malignancy. Flamen and colleagues[118] also found that FDG PET/CT scanning provided information that was additional to that obtained with conventional surveillance methods in 27% of patients. These findings could lead to changes in palliative management decisions and result in improved patient survival. Additionally, FDG PET/CT scanning can detect interval distant metastatic disease, which is seen in 8% to 17% of patients on restaging.[93] It is particularly useful in detecting new interval metastases that are either occult or difficult to diagnose prospectively on conventional imaging and is, therefore, useful in the follow-up of esophageal malignancy.[120]

NOVEL TRACERS

Although ^{18}F-FDG is the most commonly used tracer, early results using other new molecular imaging techniques have surfaced. Some of the choline derivatives that have been investigated in esophageal carcinoma include ^{11}C-choline, ^{18}F-fluoroethylcholine, and ^{18}F-fluorocholine. The advantage of these tracers is their very low uptake in normal tissues, such as brain, lung, heart, bone, and skeletal muscle. This characteristic leads to a higher signal to background ratio in malignant mediastinal adenopathy and rapid clearance from the blood after intravenous administration. The biokinetics also allow for image acquisition as early as 2 to 3 minutes after radiotracer injection.[121,122] Choline PET/CT scanning was compared with FDG PET/CT scanning in a recent study involving various tumor types. A high correlation in differentiating malignant from benign lesions based on uptake values found.[123] However, ^{11}C-choline has a short half-life of 20 minutes, limiting its use to facilities with an onsite cyclotron. Another disadvantage is its physiologic liver uptake, which may potentially obscure the detection of metastatic disease in this region.[124]

L-[3-^{18}F]-α-methyltyrosine (FAMT) is an amino acid PET tracer that is accumulated in tumor cells via an amino acid transport system, LAT-1, and is particularly important in SCC. In esophageal SCC, FAMT PET/CT imaging demonstrated lower sensitivity for lymph node staging than FDG PET/CT imaging (40% and 47%, respectively), but significantly higher specificity (100% and 50%, respectively).[125] It could even show better delineation of neoplastic disease near the heart, because FAMT lacks intense cardiac physiologic uptake commonly seen on FDG PET images. The treatment outcomes in SCC using FAMT PET/CT uptake has been studied by Sohda and colleagues.[126] When the survival rate was analyzed using a peak SUV of 2.2, uptakes values were found to correlate significantly with disease-free survival ($P = .023$).

^{18}F-fluorothymidine (FLT) is another PET tracer that reflects cellular proliferation and seems to be more specific than FDG for differentiating malignancy from inflammation.[127] This ability to differentiate malignancy from inflammation was suggested by Yue and colleagues,[127] who measured tumor cell proliferation during radiotherapy on patients with inoperable SCC. They found that, among the patients who completed radiotherapy without interruption, the parameters reflecting FLT uptake in the tumor (ie, SUV_{max} and proliferation target volume) decreased steadily whereas there was high FDG uptake in these cases. Pathologic examination of these regions revealed inflammatory infiltrates but no residual tumor. In contrast, in patients whose radiotherapy course was interrupted, FLT uptake was greater after the interruption than before the interruption. They thus concluded that FLT uptake can be used to monitor the biologic response of esophageal SCC to radiotherapy. In esophageal SCC, FLT has shown lower sensitivity but higher specificity for detection of lymph node metastatic disease as compared with FDG.[63] Although several tracers are still being assessed in clinical trails, FDG remains the most widely clinically used agent for esophageal cancer evaluation.

NOVEL PET METRICS: TEXTURAL ANALYSIS

Intratumor metabolic heterogeneity in solid tumors is reflected in their FDG uptake and distribution.[128] Texture analysis is an emerging tool to quantify the SUV heterogeneity in PET scans[129] and has been shown to predict tumor response to therapy accurately.[80,130,131] Tixier and colleagues[80] reported that intratumor texture features on pretreatment examinations can predict treatment response in esophageal cancer accurately. In another investigation by Tan and colleagues,[130] several spatial-temporal features, including SUV intensity distribution, spatial patterns (texture), tumor geometry, and associated changes resulting from CRT,

were found to be useful predictors of pathologic tumor response to neoadjuvant CRT in esophageal cancer. Reduction in SUV_{max}, decrease in SUV_{mean}, skewness, and 3 texture features (inertia, correlation, and cluster prominence) were found to be significant predictors. Additionally, a tumor was more likely to be a treatment responder in several situations: when the SUV_{mean} reduction was larger, when there were relatively fewer voxels with higher SUV values before CRT, or when FDG uptake after CRT was relatively homogeneous. Thus, longitudinal patterns in the change of metabolic activity distribution within a tumor resulting from CRT provide important information. SUV changes at the voxel level were shown to correlate well with the standard RECIST-based response assessment in metastatic colorectal cancer by Necib and colleagues.[132]

A support vector machine model, which uses several spatial-temporal PET features to characterize tumor intensity and geometry changes resulting from CRT, was constructed by Zhang and colleagues.[131] They found that this mathematical model achieved a very high rate of accuracy with a sensitivity and specificity of 100%, which was significantly better than traditional SUV measures, clinical parameters, and demographics, for predicting pathologic response in esophagus cancer. Several complex mathematical models have been developed to quantify intratumor heterogeneity with textural features of the spatial relationship between multiple image voxels extracted from FDG-PET images.[133] In another study, histograms were used to describe tumor SUV heterogeneity, and to characterize the SUV longitudinal pattern induced by CRT.[134] A greater histogram distance indicated that the tumor had been more affected by CRT. These proposed features, especially those based on the cross-bin distances, had greater accuracy than the conventional SUV values, such as SUV_{max}, SUV_{peak}, and TLG, for the prediction of pCR to CRT in esophageal cancer.

SUMMARY

Esophageal carcinoma commonly has poor outcomes, which therefore necessitates early diagnosis and treatment. Despite FDG PET/CT scanning having a limited role in the detection of early staged disease, it has been shown to be a useful tool for many reasons in patient management for esophageal carcinoma patients. There has been an impact in avoiding unnecessary interventions, as FDG PET/CT scanning has been shown to be more sensitive in detecting sites of distant metastatic disease than EUS and CT imaging. FDG PET/CT scanning has also been shown to have prognostic value in patient outcomes and monitoring treatment response. Given future radiotracer development and implementation, further investigation is needed regarding the role of molecular imaging and its place in clinical and diagnostic medicine.

REFERENCES

1. Global Burden of Disease Cancer Collaboration, Fitzmaurice C, Dicker D, Pain A, et al. The global burden of cancer 2013. JAMA Oncol 2015;1(4): 505–27.
2. Arnold M, Soerjomataram I, Ferlay J. Global incidence of oesophageal cancer by histological subtype in 2012. Gut 2015;64(3):381–7.
3. Hur C, Miller M, Kong CY, et al. Trends in esophageal adenocarcinoma incidence and mortality. Cancer 2013;119:1149–59.
4. Rustgi AK, El-Serag HB. Esophageal carcinoma. N Engl J Med 2014;371(26):2499–509.
5. Peery AF, Crockett SD, Barritt AS, et al. Burden of gastrointestinal, liver, and pancreatic diseases in the United States. Gastroenterology 2015;149(7): 1731–41.
6. Pusung M, Zeki S, Fitzgerald R. Genomics of esophageal cancer and biomarkers for early detection. Adv Exp Med Biol 2016;908:237–63.
7. Song Y, Li L, Ou Y, et al. Identification of genomic alterations in oesophageal squamous cell cancer. Nature 2014;509:91–5.
8. Zhang L, Zhou Y, Cheng C, et al. Genomic analyses reveal mutational signatures and frequently altered genes in esophageal squamous cell carcinoma. Am J Hum Genet 2015;96:597–611.
9. Bass AJ, Watanabe H, Mermel CH, et al. SOX2 is an amplified lineage-survival oncogene in lung and esophageal squamous cell carcinomas. Nat Genet 2009;41:1238–42.
10. Garraway LA, Sellers WR. Lineage dependency and lineage-survival oncogenes in human cancer. Nat Rev Cancer 2006;6:593–602.
11. Zhang W, Zhu H, Liu X, et al. Epidermal growth factor receptor is a prognosis predictor in patients with esophageal squamous cell carcinoma. Ann Thorac Surg 2014;98:513–9.
12. Gao Z, Meng X, Mu D, et al. Prognostic significance of epidermal growth factor receptor in locally advanced esophageal squamous cell carcinoma for patients receiving chemoradiotherapy. Oncol Lett 2014;7:1118–22.
13. Lagergren J, Bergstrom R, Lindgren A, et al. Symptomatic gastroesophageal reflux as a risk factor for esophageal adenocarcinoma. N Engl J Med 1999; 340:825–31.
14. Chandrasoma P, Wickramasinghe K, Ma Y, et al. Is intestinal metaplasia a necessary precursor lesion

for adenocarcinomas of the distal esophagus, gastroesophageal junction and gastric cardia? Dis Esophagus 2007;20:36–41.
15. Ek WE, Levine DM, D'Amato M, et al. Germline genetic contributions to risk for esophageal adenocarcinoma, Barrett's esophagus, and gastroesophageal reflux. J Natl Cancer Inst 2013;105:1711–8.
16. Su Z, Gay LJ, Strange A, et al. Common variants at the MHC locus and at chromosome 16q24.1 predispose to Barrett's esophagus. Nat Genet 2012; 44:1131–6.
17. Palles C, Chegwidden L, Li X, et al. Polymorphisms near TBX5 and GDF7 are associated with increased risk for Barrett's esophagus. Gastroenterology 2015;148:367–78.
18. Levine DM, Ek WE, Zhang R, et al. A genome-wide association study identifies new susceptibility loci for esophageal adenocarcinoma and Barrett's esophagus. Nat Genet 2013;45:1487–93.
19. Ismail A, Bandla S, Reveiller M, et al. Early G(1) cyclin-dependent kinases as prognostic markers and potential therapeutic targets in esophageal adenocarcinoma. Clin Cancer Res 2011;17(13): 4513–22.
20. Lin L, Bass AJ, Lockwood WW, et al. Activation of GATA binding protein 6 (GATA6) sustains oncogenic lineage-survival in esophageal adenocarcinoma. Proc Natl Acad Sci U S A 2012;109(11): 4251–6.
21. Agrawal N, Jiao Y, Bettegowda C, et al. Comparative genomic analysis of esophageal adenocarcinoma and squamous cell carcinoma. Cancer Discov 2012;2:899–905.
22. Dulak AM, Stojanov P, Peng S, et al. Exome and whole-genome sequencing of esophageal adenocarcinoma identifies recurrent driver events and mutational complexity. Nat Genet 2013;45:478–86.
23. Dulak AM, Schumacher SE, van Lieshout J, et al. Gastrointestinal adenocarcinomas of the esophagus, stomach, and colon exhibit distinct patterns of genome instability and oncogenesis. Cancer Res 2012;72:4383–93.
24. Streppel MM, Lata S, DelaBastide M, et al. Next-generation sequencing of endoscopic biopsies identifies ARID1A as a tumor-suppressor gene in Barrett's esophagus. Oncogene 2014;33(3): 347–57.
25. Schneider PM, Casson AG, Levin B, et al. Mutations of p53 in Barrett's esophagus and Barrett's cancer: a prospective study of ninety-eight cases. J Thorac Cardiovasc Surg 1996;11:323–31.
26. Barrett MT, Sanchez CA, Prevo LJ, et al. Evolution of neoplastic cell lineages in Barrett oesophagus. Nat Genet 1999;22:106–9.
27. Feber A, Xi L, Luketich JD, et al. MicroRNA expression profiles of esophageal cancer. J Thorac Cardiovasc Surg 2008;135(2):255–60.

28. Garman KS, Owzar K, Hauser ER, et al. MicroRNA expression differentiates squamous epithelium from Barrett's esophagus and esophageal cancer. Dig Dis Sci 2013;58(11):3178–88.

29. Revilla-Nuin B, Parrilla P, Lozano JJ, et al. Predictive value of MicroRNAs in the progression of Barrett esophagus to adenocarcinoma in a long-term follow-up study. Ann Surg 2013;257(5):886–93.

30. Alvi MA, Liu X, O'Donovan M, et al. DNA methylation as an adjunct to histopathology to detect prevalent, inconspicuous dysplasia and early-stage neoplasia in Barrett's esophagus. Clin Cancer Res 2013;19(4):878–88.

31. Eads CA, Lord RV, Wickramasinghe K, et al. Epigenetic patterns in the progression of esophageal adenocarcinoma. Cancer Res 2001;61(8):3410–8.

32. Wong DJ, Paulson TG, Prevo LJ, et al. p16(INK4a) lesions are common, early abnormalities that undergo clonal expansion in Barrett's metaplastic epithelium. Cancer Res 2001;61(22):8284–9.

33. Bian YS, Osterheld MC, Fontolliet C, et al. p16 inactivation by methylation of the CDKN2A promoter occurs early during neoplastic progression in Barrett's esophagus. Gastroenterology 2002;122(4):1113–21.

34. Kawakami K, Brabender J, Lord RV, et al. Hypermethylated APC DNA in plasma and prognosis of patients with esophageal adenocarcinoma. J Natl Cancer Inst 2000;92(22):1805–11.

35. Bongiorno PF, al-Kasspooles M, Lee SW, et al. E-cadherin expression in primary and metastatic thoracic neoplasms and in Barrett's oesophagus. Br J Cancer 1995;71(1):166–72.

36. Peters CJ, Rees JR, Hardwick RH, et al. A 4-gene signature predicts survival of patients with resected adenocarcinoma of the esophagus, junction, and gastric cardia. Gastroenterology 2010; 139:1995–2004.

37. Kim SM, Park YY, Park ES, et al. Prognostic biomarkers for esophageal adenocarcinoma identified by analysis of tumor transcriptome. PLoS One 2010;5(11):e15074.

38. Ong CA, Shapiro J, Nason KS, et al. Three-gene immunohistochemical panel adds to clinical staging algorithms to predict prognosis for patients with esophageal adenocarcinoma. J Clin Oncol 2013;31:1576–82.

39. Schauer M, Janssen KP, Rimkus C, et al. Microarray-based response prediction in esophageal adenocarcinoma. Clin Cancer Res 2010;16:330–7.

40. Lagarde SM, Ver Loren van Themaat PE, Moerland PD, et al. Analysis of gene expression identifies differentially expressed genes and pathways associated with lymphatic dissemination in patients with adenocarcinoma of the esophagus. Ann Surg Oncol 2008;15:3459–70.

41. Goh XY, Rees JR, Paterson AL, et al. Integrative analysis of array-comparative genomic hybridisation and matched gene expression profiling data reveals novel genes with prognostic significance in oesophageal adenocarcinoma. Gut 2011;60:1317–26.

42. Rice TW, Ishwaran H, Ferguson MK, et al. Cancer of the esophagus and esophagogastric junction: an eighth edition staging primer. J Thorac Oncol 2017;12:36–42.

43. Rice TW, Kelsen DP, Blackstone EH, et al. Esophagus and esophagogastric junction. In: Amin MB, Edge SB, Greene FL, editors. AJCC cancer staging manual. 8th edition. New York: Springer; 2017. p. 185–202.

44. Ajani JA, Barthel JS, Bentrem DJ, et al. Esophageal and esophagogastric junction cancers clinical practice guidelines in oncology. J Natl Compr Canc Netw 2011;9:830–87.

45. Alsop BR, Sharma P. Esophageal cancer. Gastroenterol Clin North Am 2016;45(3):399–412.

46. Elsadek HM, Radwan MM. Diagnostic accuracy of mucosal biopsy versus endoscopic mucosal resection in Barrett's esophagus and related superficial lesions. Int Sch Res Notices 2015;2015: 735807.

47. Walker AJ, Spier BJ, Perlman SB, et al. Integrated PET/CT fusion imaging and endoscopic ultrasound in the pre-operative staging and evaluation of esophageal cancer. Mol Imaging Biol 2011;13: 166–71.

48. Muijs CT, Beukema JC, Pruim J, et al. A systematic review on the role of FDG-PET/CT in tumour delineation and radiotherapy planning in patients with esophageal cancer. Radiother Oncol 2010;97: 165–71.

49. Shi W, Wang W, Wang J, et al. Meta-analysis of 18FDG PET-CT for nodal staging in patients with esophageal cancer. Surg Oncol 2013;22: 112–6.

50. Smyth EC, Shah MA. Role of [18]F 2-fluoro-2-deoxyglucose positron emission tomography in upper gastrointestinal malignancies. World J Gastroenterol 2011;17:5059–74.

51. Varghese TK, Hofstetter WL, Rizk NP, et al. The Society of thoracic surgery guidelines on the diagnosis and staging of patients with esophageal cancer. Ann Thorac Surg 2013;96:346–56.

52. van Westreenen HL, Westerterp M, Bossuyt PM, et al. Systematic review of the staging performance of 18F-fluorodeoxyglucose positron emission tomography in esophageal cancer. J Clin Oncol 2004;22:3805–12.

53. Meyers BF, Downey RJ, Decker PA, et al, American College of Surgeons Oncology Group Z0060. The utility of positron emission tomography in staging of potentially operable carcinoma of the thoracic esophagus: results of the American College of Surgeons Oncology Group Z0060 trial. J Thorac Cardiovasc Surg 2007;133:738–45.

54. Barber TW, Duong CP, Leong T, et al. 18F-FDG PET/CT has a high impact on patient management and provides powerful prognostic stratification in the primary staging of esophageal cancer: a prospective study with mature survival data. J Nucl Med 2012;53:864–71.

55. Gillies RS, Middleton MR, Maynard ND, et al. Additional benefit of ^{18}F-fluorodeoxyglucose integrated positron emission tomography/computed tomography in the staging of oesophageal cancer. Eur Radiol 2011;21:274–80.

56. Blencowe NS, Whistance RN, Strong S, et al. Evaluating the role of fluorodeoxyglucose positron emission tomography-computed tomography in multi-disciplinary team recommendations for oesophago-gastric cancer. Br J Cancer 2013;109: 1445–50.

57. Foley KG, Lewis WG, Fielding P, et al. N-staging of oesophageal and junctional carcinoma: is there still a role for EUS in patients staged N0 at PET/CT? Clin Radiol 2014;69:959–64.

58. Pech O, May A, Manner H, et al. Long-term efficacy and safety of endoscopic resection for patients with mucosal adenocarcinoma of the esophagus. Gastroenterology 2014;146:652–60.

59. Moon SH, Kim HS, Hyun SH, et al. Prediction of occult lymph node metastasis by metabolic parameters in patients with clinically N0 esophageal squamous cell carcinoma. J Nucl Med 2014;55: 743–8.

60. Blank S, Lordick F, Dobritz M, et al. A reliable risk score for stage IV esophagogastric cancer. Eur J Surg Oncol 2013;39:823–30.

61. Stahl M, Mariette C, Haustermans K, et al. Oesophageal cancer: ESMO Clinical Practice Guidelines for diagnosis, treatment and follow-up. Ann Oncol 2013;24(Suppl 6):vi51–6.

62. You JJ, Wong RK, Darling G, et al. Clinical utility of 18F-fluorodeoxyglucose positron emission tomography/computed tomography in the staging of patients with potentially resectable esophageal cancer. J Thorac Oncol 2013;8:1563–9.

63. Han D, Yu J, Zhong X, et al. Comparison of the diagnostic value of 3-deoxy-3-18F-fluorothymidine and 18F-fluorodeoxyglucose positron emission tomography/computed tomography in the assessment of regional lymph node in thoracic esophageal squamous cell carcinoma: a pilot study. Dis Esophagus 2012;25:416–26.

64. Yamamoto Y, Nishiyama Y, Ishikawa S, et al. Correlation of 18F-FLT and 18F-FDG uptake on PET with Ki-67 immunohistochemistry in non-small cell lung cancer. Eur J Nucl Med Mol Imaging 2007;34: 1610–6.

65. Rizk N, Downey RJ, Akhurst T, et al. Preoperative 18[F]-fluorodeoxyglucose positron emission tomography standardized uptake values predict survival after esophageal adenocarcinoma resection. Ann Thorac Surg 2006;81:1076–81.

66. Cerfolio RJ, Bryant AS. Maximum standardized uptake values on positron emission tomography of esophageal cancer predicts stage, tumor biology, and survival. Ann Thorac Surg 2006;82:391–4.

67. Ott K, Weber WA, Lordick F, et al. Metabolic imaging predicts response, survival, and recurrence in adenocarcinomas of the esophagogastric junction. J Clin Oncol 2006;24:4692–8.

68. Pan L, Gu P, Huang G, et al. Prognostic significance of SUV on PET/CT in patients with esophageal cancer: a systematic review and meta-analysis. Eur J Gastroenterol Hepatol 2009;21:1008–15.

69. Westerterp M, Sloof GW, Hoekstra OS, et al. [18]FDG uptake in oesophageal adenocarcinoma: linking biology and outcome. J Cancer Res Clin Oncol 2008;134:227–36.

70. Omloo JM, van Heijl M, Hoekstra OS, et al. FDG-PET parameters as prognostic factor in esophageal cancer patients: a review. Ann Surg Oncol 2011;18:3338–52.

71. Omloo JM, Westerterp M, Sloof GW, et al. The value of positron emission tomography in the diagnosis and treatment of oesophageal cancer. Ned Tijdschr Geneeskd 2008;152:365–70 [in Dutch].

72. Choi JY, Janq HJ, Shim YM, et al. 18F-FDG PET in patients with esophageal squamous cell carcinoma undergoing curative surgery: prognostic implications. J Nucl Med 2004;45:1843–50.

73. Kato H, Takita J, Miyazaki T, et al. Correlation of 18-F-fluorodeoxyglucose (FDG) accumulation with glucose transporter (Glut-1) expression in esophageal squamous cell carcinoma. Anticancer Res 2003;23:3263–72.

74. Kleespies A, Guba M, Jauch KW, et al. Vascular endothelial growth factor in esophageal cancer. J Surg Oncol 2004;87:95–104.

75. Schreurs LM, Smit JK, Pavlov K, et al. Prognostic impact of clinicopathological features and expression of biomarkers related to (18)F-FDG uptake in esophageal cancer. Ann Surg Oncol 2014;21: 3751–7.

76. Hsu PK, Lin KH, Wang SJ, et al. Pre-operative positron emission tomography/computed tomography predicts advanced lymph node metastasis in esophageal squamous cell carcinoma patients. World J Surg 2011;35:1321–6, 29.

77. Hsu WH, Hsu PK, Wang SJ, et al. Positron emission tomography-computed tomography in predicting locoregional invasion in esophageal squamous cell carcinoma. Ann Thorac Surg 2009;87:1564–8.

78. Wahl RL, Jacene H, Kasamon Y, et al. From RECIST to PERCIST: evolving considerations for PET response criteria in solid tumors. J Nucl Med 2009;50:122S–50S.

79. El Naqa I, Grigsby P, Apte A, et al. Exploring feature-based approaches in PET images for predicting cancer treatment outcomes. Pattern Recognit 2009;42:1162–71.

80. Tixier F, Le Rest CC, Hatt M, et al. Intratumor heterogeneity characterized by textural features on baseline ^{18}F-FDG PET images predicts response to concomitant radiochemotherapy in esophageal cancer. J Nucl Med 2011;52:369–78.

81. Hyun SH, Choi JY, Shim YM, et al. Prognostic value of metabolic tumor volume measured by 18F-fluorodeoxyglucose positron emission tomography in patients with esophageal carcinoma. Ann Surg Oncol 2010;17:115–22.

82. Malik V, Johnston C, O'Toole D, et al. Metabolic tumor volume provides complementary prognostic information to EUS staging in esophageal and junctional cancer. Dis Esophagus 2017;30(3):1–8.

83. Li YM, Lin Q, Zhao L, et al. Pre-treatment metabolic tumor volume and total lesion glycolysis are useful prognostic factors for esophageal squamous cell cancer patients. Asian Pac J Cancer Prev 2014; 15:1369–73.

84. Fiorica F, di Bona D, Schepis F, et al. Preoperative chemoradiotherapy for oesophageal cancer: a systematic review and meta-analysis. Gut 2004;53: 925–30.

85. Jin HL, Zhu H, Ling TS, et al. Neoadjuvant chemoradiotherapy for resectable esophageal carcinoma: a meta-analysis. World J Gastroenterol 2009;15:5983–91.

86. Urba SG, Orringer MB, Turrisi A, et al. Randomized trial of preoperative chemoradiation versus surgery alone in patients with locoregional esophageal carcinoma. J Clin Oncol 2001;19:305–13.

87. Meredith KL, Weber JM, Turaga KK, et al. Pathologic response after neoadjuvant therapy is the major determinant of survival in patients with esophageal cancer. Ann Surg Oncol 2010;17: 1159–67.

88. Dittrick GW, Weber JM, Shridhar R, et al. Pathologic nonresponders after neoadjuvant chemoradiation for esophageal cancer demonstrate no survival benefit compared with patients treated with primary esophagectomy. Ann Surg Oncol 2012;19:1678–84.

89. Hsu PK, Chien LI, Huang CS, et al. Comparison of survival among neoadjuvant chemoradiation responders, non-responders and patients receiving primary resection for locally advanced oesophageal squamous cell carcinoma: does neoadjuvant chemoradiation benefit all? Interact Cardiovasc Thorac Surg 2013;17:460–6.

90. Heger U, Bader F, Lordick F, et al. Interim endoscopy results during neoadjuvant therapy for gastric cancer correlate with histopathological response and prognosis. Gastric Cancer 2014;17:478–88.

91. Blank S, Lordick F, Bader F, et al. Post-therapeutic response evaluation by a combination of endoscopy and CT scan in esophagogastric adenocarcinoma after chemotherapy: better than its reputation. Gastric Cancer 2015;18(2):314–25.

92. Westerterp M, van Westreenen HL, Reitsma JB, et al. Esophageal cancer: CT, endoscopic US, and FDG PET for assessment of response to neoadjuvant therapy– systematic review. Radiology 2005;236:841–51.

93. Kim TJ, Kim HY, Lee KW, et al. Multimodality assessment of esophageal cancer: preoperative staging and monitoring of response to therapy. Radiographics 2009;29:403–21.

94. Tirkes T, Hollar MA, Tann M, et al. Response criteria in oncologic imaging: review of traditional and new criteria. Radiographics 2013;33:1323–41.

95. Yanagawa M, Tatsumi M, Miyata H, et al. Evaluation of response to neoadjuvant chemotherapy for esophageal cancer: PET response criteria in solid tumors versus response evaluation criteria in solid tumors. J Nucl Med 2012;53:872–80.

96. Molena D, Sun HH, Badr AS, et al. Clinical tools do not predict pathological complete response in patients with esophageal squamous cell cancer treated with definitive chemoradiotherapy. Dis Esophagus 2014;27:355–9.

97. Cerfolio RJ, Bryant AS, Talati AA, et al. Change in maximum standardized uptake value on repeat positron emission tomography after chemoradiotherapy in patients with esophageal cancer identifies complete responders. J Thorac Cardiovasc Surg 2009;137:605–9.

98. Yen TJ, Chung CS, Wu YW, et al. Comparative study between endoscopic ultrasonography and positron emission tomography-computed tomography in staging patients with esophageal squamous cell carcinoma. Dis Esophagus 2012;25:40–7.

99. Port JL, Lee PC, Korst RJ, et al. Positron emission tomographic scanning predicts survival after induction chemotherapy for esophageal carcinoma. Ann Thorac Surg 2007;84:393–400 [discussion: 400].

100. Kim MK, Ryu JS, Kim SB, et al. Value of complete metabolic response by (18)F-fluorodeoxyglucose-positron emission tomography in oesophageal cancer for prediction of pathologic response and survival after preoperative chemoradiotherapy. Eur J Cancer 2007;43:1385–91.

101. Erasmus JJ, Munden RF, Truong MT, et al. Preoperative chemo-radiation-induced ulceration in patients with esophageal cancer: a confounding factor in tumor response assessment in integrated computed tomographic-positron emission tomographic imaging. J Thorac Oncol 2006;1:478–86.

102. Bruzzi JF, Munden RF, Truong MT, et al. PET/CT of esophageal cancer: its role in clinical management. Radiographics 2007;27:1635–52.

103. Krause BJ, Herrmann K, Wieder H, et al. 18F-FDG PET and 18F-FDG PET/CT for assessing response to therapy in esophageal cancer. J Nucl Med 2009;50:89S–96S.

104. Schmidt T, Lordick F, Herrmann K, et al. Value of functional imaging by PET in esophageal cancer. J Natl Compr Canc Netw 2015;13(2):239–47.

105. Weber WA, Ott K, Becker K, et al. Prediction of response to preoperative chemotherapy in adenocarcinomas of the esophagogastric junction by metabolic imaging. J Clin Oncol 2001;19:3058–65.

106. Lordick F, Ott K, Krause BJ, et al. PET to assess early metabolic response and to guide treatment of adenocarcinoma of the oesophagogastric junction: the MUNICON phase II trial. Lancet Oncol 2007;8:797–805.

107. zum Büschenfelde CM, Herrmann K, Schuster T, et al. (18)F-FDG PET-guided salvage neoadjuvant radiochemotherapy of adenocarcinoma of the esophagogastric junction: the MUNICON II trial. J Nucl Med 2011;52:1189–96.

108. van Heijl M, Omloo JM, van Berge Henegouwen MI, et al. Fluorodeoxyglucose positron emission tomography for evaluating early response during neoadjuvant chemoradiotherapy in patients with potentially curable esophageal cancer. Ann Surg 2011;253: 56–63.

109. Ilson DH, Minsky BD, Ku GY, et al. Phase 2 trial of induction and concurrent chemoradiotherapy with weekly irinotecan and cisplatin followed by surgery for esophageal cancer. Cancer 2012;118:2820–7.

110. Wieder HA, Brücher BL, Zimmermann F, et al. Time course of tumor metabolic activity during chemoradiotherapy of esophageal squamous cell carcinoma and response to treatment. J Clin Oncol 2004;22:900–8.

111. Chao KS. Functional imaging for early prediction of response to chemoradiotherapy: 3'-deoxy-3'-18F-fluorothymidine positron emission tomography–a clinical application model of esophageal cancer. Semin Oncol 2006;33:S59–63.

112. Apisarnthanarax S, Alauddin MM, Mourtada F, et al. Early detection of chemoradioresponse in esophageal carcinoma by 3'-deoxy-3'-3H-fluorothymidine using preclinical tumor models. Clin Cancer Res 2006;12:4590–7.

113. Benz MR, Herrmann K, Walter F, et al. (18)F-FDG PET/CT for monitoring treatment responses to the epidermal growth factor receptor inhibitor erlotinib. J Nucl Med 2011;52(11):1684–9.

114. Mileshkin L, Hicks RJ, Hughes BG, et al. Changes in 18F-fluorodeoxyglucose and 18F-fluorodeoxythymidine positron emission tomography imaging in patients with non-small cell lung cancer treated with erlotinib. Clin Cancer Res 2011;17(10):3304–15.

115. Downey RJ, Akhurst T, Ilson D, et al. Whole body 18FDG-PET and the response of esophageal cancer to induction therapy: results of a prospective trial. J Clin Oncol 2003;21:428–32.

116. Schollaert P, Crott R, Bertrand C, et al. A systematic review of the predictive value of (18)FDG-PET in esophageal and esophagogastric junction cancer after neoadjuvant chemoradiation on the survival outcome stratification. J Gastrointest Surg 2014;18: 894–905.

117. Kwee RM. Prediction of tumor response to neoadjuvant therapy in patients with esophageal cancer with use of 18F FDG PET: a systematic review. Radiology 2010;254:707–17.

118. Flamen P, Lerut A, Van Cutsem E, et al. The utility of positron emission tomography for the diagnosis and staging of recurrent esophageal cancer. J Thorac Cardiovasc Surg 2000;120:1085–92.

119. Cerfolio RJ, Bryant AS, Ohja B, et al. The accuracy of endoscopic ultrasonography with fine-needle aspiration, integrated positron emission tomography with computed tomography, and computed tomography in restaging patients with esophageal cancer after neoadjuvant chemoradiotherapy. J Thorac Cardiovasc Surg 2005;129:1232–41.

120. Bruzzi JF, Swisher SG, Truong MT, et al. Detection of interval distant metastases: clinical utility of integrated CT-PET imaging in patients with esophageal carcinoma after neoadjuvant therapy. Cancer 2007;109:125–34.

121. DeGrado TR, Baldwin SW, Wang S, et al. Synthesis and evaluation of 18F-labeled choline analogs as oncologic PET tracers. J Nucl Med 2001;42: 1805–14.

122. Hara T. 18F-fluorocholine: a new oncologic PET tracer. J Nucl Med 2001;42:1815–7.

123. Tian M, Zhang H, Higuchi T, et al. Oncological diagnosis using (11)C-choline-positron emission tomography in comparison with 2-deoxy-2-[(18)F] fluoro-D-glucose-positron emission tomography. Mol Imaging Biol 2004;6:172–9.

124. Kwee SA, DeGrado TR, Talbot JN, et al. Cancer imaging with fluorine-18-labeled choline derivatives. Semin Nucl Med 2007;37:420–8.

125. Sohda M, Kato H, Suzuki S, et al. 18F-FAMT-PET is useful for the diagnosis of lymph node metastasis in operable esophageal squamous cell carcinoma. Ann Surg Oncol 2010;17:3181–6.

126. Sohda M, Sakai M, Honjyo H. Use of pre-treatment 18F-FAMT PET to predict patient survival in squamous cell carcinoma of the esophagus treated by curative surgery. Anticancer Res 2014;34(7): 3623–8.

127. Yue J, Chen L, Cabrera AR, et al. Measuring tumor cell proliferation with 18F-FLT PET during radiotherapy of esophageal squamous cell carcinoma: a pilot clinical study. J Nucl Med 2010;51:528–34.

128. Zhao S, Kuge Y, Mochizuki T, et al. Biologic correlates of intratumoral heterogeneity in ^{18}F-FDG

distribution with regional expression of glucose transporters and hexokinase-II in experimental tumor. J Nucl Med 2005;46:675–82.

129. Chicklore S, Goh V, Siddique M, et al. Cook, quantifying tumour heterogeneity in (18)F-FDG PET/CT imaging by texture analysis. Eur J Nucl Med Mol Imaging 2013;40:133–40.

130. Tan S, Kligerman S, Chen W, et al. Spatial-temporal [18F] FDG-PET features for predicting pathologic response of esophageal cancer to neoadjuvant chemoradiation therapy. Int J Radiat Oncol Biol Phys 2013;85:1375–82.

131. Zhang H, Tan S, Chen W, et al. Modeling pathologic response of locally advanced esophageal cancer to chemoradiotherapy using spatial-temporal FDG-PET features, clinical parameters and demographics. Int J Radiat Oncol Biol Phys 2014;88(1):195–203.

132. Necib H, Garcia C, Wagner A, et al. Detection and characterization of tumor changes in ^{18}F-FDG PET patient monitoring using parametric imaging. J Nucl Med 2011;52:354–61.

133. Rahim M, Kim S, So H, et al. Recent trends in PET image interpretations using volumetric and texture-based quantification methods in nuclear oncology. Nucl Med Mol Imaging 2014;48:1–15.

134. Tan S, Zhang H, Zhang Y, et al. Predicting pathologic tumor response to chemoradiotherapy with histogram distances characterizing longitudinal changes in 18F-FDG uptake patterns. Med Phys 2013;40(10):101707.

Molecular Imaging and Precision Medicine in Uterine and Ovarian Cancers

 CrossMark

Katherine A. Zukotynski, MD, FRCPC[a,b,*], Chun K. Kim, MD[c]

KEYWORDS

- Uterine cancer • Endometrial cancer • Cervical cancer • Ovarian cancer • Gynecologic malignancy
- Positron emission tomography • Cancer staging • Precision medicine

KEY POINTS

- PET is helpful to accurately stage patients with potentially curable gynecologic cancer.
- PET plays an important role in the initial treatment strategy by evaluating disease extent and assessing the molecular pathobiology so that appropriate therapy can be initiated.
- PET is helpful for developing subsequent treatment strategy in patients with gynecologic cancer including monitoring therapy response, detection of recurrence, and prediction of outcome.

INTRODUCTION: PRECISION MEDICINE AND GYNECOLOGIC CANCER

Precision medicine integrates the clinical, molecular pathobiology, and genetic picture of a disease to diagnose, stage, provide predictive and prognostic information of therapy response, and ultimately suggest patient outcome. The hope is that, by using precision medicine, the right treatment can be given to the right patient at the right time, while expensive, toxic, futile treatment can be avoided in those who will likely not respond. Gynecologic cancer is a heterogeneous group of diseases both functionally and morphologically, typically classified according to the anatomic site of origin.[1] Anatomic imaging with ultrasound (US), computed tomography (CT), and MR imaging has long been used in clinical practice to evaluate patients with gynecologic malignancy. More recently, the addition of metabolic imaging with

PET has been shown to provide insight into the biologic behavior and extent of disease to guide therapy selection.[2–7] The annual report of the United States National Oncology PET Registry indicated that approximately 10% of all PET studies were performed to evaluate patients with gynecologic cancer and that, in 38% of cases, the results led to a change in treatment strategy, emphasizing the usefulness of PET.[7]

There are several PET radiotracers, the most common of which is ^{18}F-labeled 2-fluoro-2-deoxy-D-glucose (FDG), a radioactive glucose analogue that is helpful to detect tumor glucose metabolism throughout the body and monitor early therapy response. As with other cancer types, FDG uptake depends on several factors, such as cellular histology, density, aggressiveness, and technical parameters. Standardized technique is important for reproducible results, and several

The authors have nothing to disclose.
[a] Division of Nuclear Medicine and Molecular Imaging, Department of Medicine, McMaster University, 1200 Main Street West, Hamilton, Ontario L8S 4L8, Canada; [b] Division of Nuclear Medicine and Molecular Imaging, Department of Radiology, McMaster University, 1200 Main Street West, Hamilton, Ontario L8S 4L8, Canada; [c] Division of Nuclear Medicine and Molecular Imaging, Department of Radiology, Brigham and Women's Hospital, Harvard Medical School, 75 Francis Street, Boston, MA 02492, USA
* Corresponding author. Division of Nuclear Medicine and Molecular Imaging, Department of Medicine, McMaster University, 1200 Main Street West, Hamilton, Ontario L8S 4L8, Canada.
E-mail address: katherine.zukotynski@utoronto.ca

pet.theclinics.com

studies have evaluated metabolic parameters, such as the intensity of tumor FDG uptake or standardized uptake value (SUV) across different scanner types.[8,9] Results in the literature have found equivalence between PET image quality, lesion detection rate, and a high correlation between SUV derived from PET/CT and PET/MR imaging.[10,11]

Additional PET radiotracers may be of benefit in gynecologic cancer, including 3'-deoxy-3'-[^{18}F] fluorothymidine,[12,13] ^{60}Cu-labeled diacetyl-bis (N4-methylthiosemicarbazone)[14] and 16α-[^{18}F]-fluoro-17β-estradiol (FES),[15] among others. Richard and colleagues[12] showed an increasing trend between 3'-deoxy-3'-[^{18}F] fluorothymidine uptake and Ki67 mitotic index in a pilot study of 6 women with suspected new and recurrent ovarian carcinoma. Dehdashti and colleagues[16] studied tumor hypoxia using ^{60}Cu-labeled diacetyl-bis (N4-methylthiosemicarbazone) PET in a group of 14 women with biopsy-proven cervical cancer and its association with response to radiotherapy and chemotherapy. The study concluded that tumor ^{60}Cu-labeled diacetyl-bis (N4-methylthiosemicarbazone) uptake was related inversely to progression-free survival and overall survival, and could be used to discriminate those patients likely to develop recurrence after therapy. Tsujikawa and colleagues[15] studied the correlation between estrogen receptor expression, glucose metabolism, and the clinicopathologic features of endometrial tumors. The study was based on the premise that, as endometrial carcinoma progresses to higher stage and grade, so too does it have reduced estrogen dependence and accelerated glucose metabolism. In a sample of 22 patients with endometrial cancer and 9 with endometrial hyperplasia, it was shown that high-risk carcinoma had a significantly higher FDG to FES SUV ratio than low-risk carcinoma and low-risk carcinoma had a significantly higher FDG to FES SUV ratio than endometrial hyperplasia. It was concluded that use of an FDG to FES SUV ratio could noninvasively assess the molecular makeup of endometrial carcinoma and suggest the effectiveness of targeted hormonal therapy.

In general, the literature suggests that, through the use of different PET probes, the regional heterogeneous signature of gynecologic cancer, including differences in cellular proliferation, hypoxia, and estrogen receptor expression, can be studied and may be of help in understanding tumor biology and predicting outcome. Although clinical trials conducted to date have not sought to stratify patients according to the molecular basis of disease, based on the studies available, we are at the cusp of being able to use targeted molecular imaging to do so. For the purposes of this article, we focus on FDG-PET/CT and PET/MR imaging in endometrial cancer, cervical cancer and ovarian cancer.

PET SCANS IN THE INITIAL TREATMENT STRATEGY OF GYNECOLOGIC MALIGNANCY
Initial Staging

Staging gynecologic malignancy relies on a combination of the International Federation of Gynecology and Obstetrics (FIGO) and TNM systems. Depending on tumor type and physician preference, a combination of clinical, surgical, and imaging findings is used to assess disease spread as well as histologic tumor type and grade.[17–20] In general, MR imaging is the preferred imaging modality to evaluate the primary site of disease and CT is the most commonly used imaging modality to detect lymph node spread and metastases.[21] The addition of PET is particularly helpful to evaluate metabolically active disease extent.[2] For staging the site of primary disease (T status), PET can pinpoint metabolically active malignant disease (**Fig. 1**). For evaluating the spread of malignant disease to the lymph nodes (N status), the principal strengths of PET include (1) detection of metabolically active metastatic disease spread to lymph nodes that seem to be structurally normal, (2) differentiation of benign from malignant enlarged lymph nodes based on abnormal metabolic activity, and (3) evaluation of the entire body (**Figs. 2–4**). One of the true strengths of PET lies in its ability to detect distant metastases (M status), to exclude a metastatic deposit in an anatomically indeterminate or suspicious lesion (**Fig. 5**) or to identify additional incidental sites of malignant disease (**Fig. 6**). Results in the literature suggest both PET/MR imaging and PET/CT play an important role in staging and have significant impact on precision management, including therapy intent (ie, cure vs palliation) and selection (ie, surgery vs radiation and chemotherapy).[5,22] Although PET/MR imaging is preferred for primary tumor delineation[22] and detection of liver metastases, particularly when liver lesions are small (<1 cm), PET/CT is preferred for the assessment of distant disease spread, particularly to bone.[2]

Endometrial cancer
Endometrial cancer is the most commonly diagnosed gynecologic malignancy in the United States, estimated to account for approximately 60,000 new cases and 10,000 deaths in 2016.[23] It is classified into 2 groups.[24] Type 1 includes

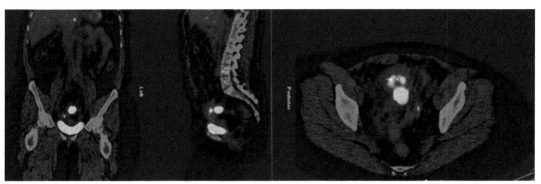

Fig. 1. Coronal, sagittal, and axial fused PET with ^{18}F-labeled 2-fluoro-2-deoxy-D-glucose (FDG)/computed tomography images show intense focal FDG uptake localizing to a site of biopsy-proven endometrial cancer. Otherwise, the scan shows no evidence of regional or distant metastatic disease.

endometrioid histology with grade 1 and 2 differentiation and is an estrogen-dependent cancer arising in the setting of endometrial hyperplasia with a good prognosis. Type II includes grade 3 endometrioid tumors and tumors with nonendometrioid histology, such as serous papillary carcinoma, clear cell–type carcinoma, or carcinosarcoma (any grade) and is a non–estrogen-dependent cancer with aggressive features, arising in an atrophic endometrial background.

Several features are considered high risk for disease spread and recurrence, including type II disease, large tumors (>2 cm), deep myometrial invasion (>50%), or cervical stromal involvement.[25–28] Prognosis depends on clinical and histopathologic factors as well as disease stage.

The majority of women with endometrial cancer present with abnormal vaginal bleeding, and are diagnosed with early stage disease after transvaginal ultrasound examination and endometrial

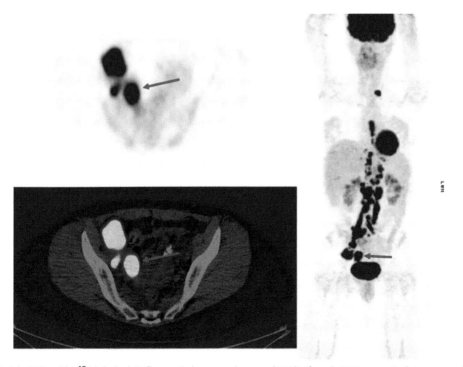

Fig. 2. Axial PET with ^{18}F-labeled 2-fluoro-2-deoxy-D-glucose (FDG), fused PET/computed tomography and maximum intensity projection images show intense FDG uptake in the right ovary (*red arrow*) at a site of ovarian cancer as well as multiple intensely FDG-avid lymph nodes in the pelvis, abdomen, mediastinum, and left supraclavicular region highly suspicious for extensive lymph node disease spread throughout the body.

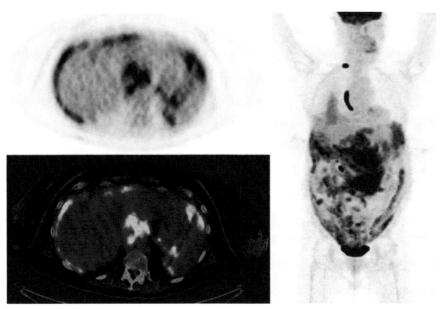

Fig. 3. Axial PET with ^{18}F-labeled 2-fluoro-2-deoxy-D-glucose (FDG), fused PET/computed tomography (CT), and maximum intensity projection images from a PET/CT scan performed on a 69-year-old woman with ovarian cancer show extensive peritoneal and mesenteric disease with FDG-avid nodal conglomerates and multiple perihepatic, perisplenic, and serosal implants. The intense FDG uptake in the right supraclavicular region and along the course of the superior vena cava was associated with a port-A-cath, and mild diffuse radiotracer uptake in the right hemithorax was associated with a pleural effusion.

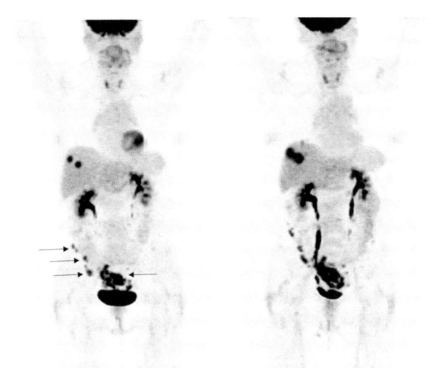

Fig. 4. Maximum intensity projection images from PET with ^{18}F-labeled 2-fluoro-2-deoxy-D-glucose (FDG)/computed tomography scans obtained before (*left*) and after (*right*) therapy in a woman with advanced ovarian cancer show intense radiotracer uptake at sites of peritoneal disease (*arrows*) and liver metastases that progressed despite therapy.

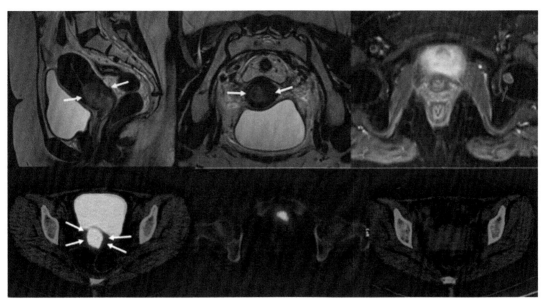

Fig. 5. Selected MR imaging and PET with ^{18}F-labeled 2-fluoro-2-deoxy-D-glucose (FDG)/computed tomography (CT) images in a 48-year-old woman with stage IIIB cervical adenocarcinoma after radiation and chemotherapy, to evaluate for possible recurrent disease. The sagittal (*upper left*) and axial (*upper middle*) MR images show a 4.6 × 2.8 × 3.2 cm mass (*yellow arrows*) centered within the cervix suspicious for recurrent disease. An enhancing lesion was also seen in the left femoral head (*red arrow*), concerning for metastasis (*upper right*). Axial fused FDG PET/CT images show intense baseline FDG uptake in the cervix consistent with recurrence (*lower left: white arrows*), but no abnormal FDG uptake in the left femoral head (*lower middle*), making metastasis very unlikely. Subsequently, the patient received chemotherapy; a midtherapy PET/CT performed after 3 cycles (*lower right*) showed complete resolution of metabolic activity, suggesting a good treatment response.

biopsy. Although localized disease may be curable, the involvement of lymph nodes and distant disease significantly impacts outcome. Indeed, the 5-year survival of endometrial cancer localized to the uterus is greater than 95%, whereas it is 57% with pelvic lymph node spread, 49% with abdominal lymph node spread, and approximately 16% with distant metastases.[23,29]

Accurate staging is key to determining appropriate therapy. The FIGO system stages endometrial cancer surgically and treatment typically includes hysterectomy with bilateral salpingo-oophorectomy unless there is distant disease spread. The uterus has a complex lymphatic drainage system and paraaortic lymph nodes may be involved without pelvic lymph nodes. Although controversial, resection of pelvic and paraaortic lymph nodes is often included at the time of staging, particularly in patients with disease at high risk for spread.[30] A multicenter, prospective, cohort study of patients with clinical stage 1 endometrial cancer suggest sentinel lymph node mapping has a high degree of diagnostic accuracy in detecting disease spread and may obviate the need for complete lymphadenectomy.[31] Also, imaging may be helpful to evaluate

disease extent, particularly in patients being considered for fertility-sparing management, patients with biopsy-proven high-risk histology, or patients with suspected extrauterine disease.[32] Although there is variability in practice among institutions, MR imaging is preferred for delineating myometrial extension, cervical stromal, uterine serosal, adnexal, vaginal, and/or parametrial involvement. PET is the imaging modality of choice for the evaluation of distant disease spread[33–36] and may obviate the need for surgery if unsuspected sites of distant metastases are detected.[37] The reported sensitivity and specificity for detecting endometrial cancer lymph node spread is: 28% to 64% (sensitivity) and 78% to 94% (specificity) for CT; 59% to 72% (sensitivity) and 93% to 97% (specificity) for MR imaging[33–36]; and 74% to 77% (sensitivity) and 93% to 100% (specificity) for PET/CT.[34–36] Sironi and colleagues[38] and Kitajima and colleagues[39] suggested the sensitivity of PET/CT depends on lymph node size, with decreased sensitivity in lymph nodes less than 5 mm in short axis diameter. Although PET may be falsely positive in patients with benign conditions, such as infection or inflammation, in general the specificity is high (>90%). However,

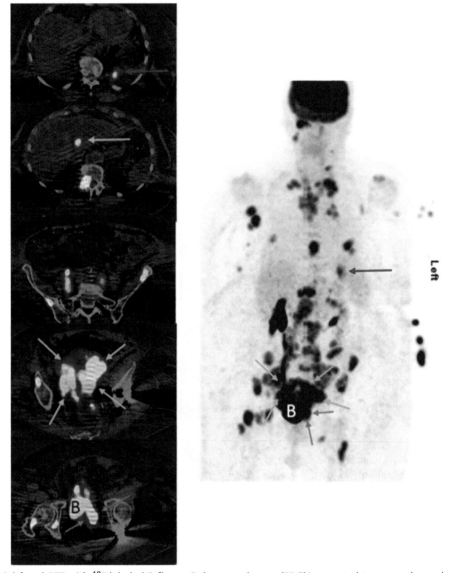

Fig. 6. Axial fused PET with ^{18}F-labeled 2-fluoro-2-deoxy-D-glucose (FDG)/computed tomography and maximum intensity projection images from a scan performed on a 78-year-old woman with vaginal bleeding and clinically suspected endometrial cancer show intensely FDG-avid endometrial (*green arrows*) and cervical masses (*orange arrows*), abdominal and pelvic lymph nodes, as well as a left supraclavicular lymph node, a liver metastasis (*blue arrows*), a left lower lobe lung metastasis (*red arrows*) with adjacent atelectasis, and numerous skeletal metastases. The patient was found to have concurrent metastatic endometrial and cervical cancer. "B" denotes the urinary bladder.

although PET improves the detection of disease spread compared with contrast enhanced diagnostic CT, the results of ACRIN 6671/GOG 0233, a prospective multicenter study conducted by the American College of Radiology Imaging Network (ACRIN) and the Gynecologic Oncology Group (GOG), published earlier this year concluded that PET/CT did not obviate the need for surgical sampling given the moderate sensitivity.[40]

Cervical cancer
Cervical cancer is a leading cause of cancer-related death in women worldwide; however, with the advent of routine screening in the developed world, the incidence and mortality has significantly decreased. In the United States, cervical cancer was estimated to account for approximately 13,000 new cases and 4000 deaths in 2016.[41] Although localized disease may be curable, involvement of the lymph nodes

significantly impacts outcome. Indeed, the 5-year survival of cancer localized to the cervix is greater than 91%, whereas it is only 57% with spread to pelvic lymph nodes and 16% when distant disease is present.[41]

Based on the FIGO classification system, cervical cancer is staged clinically. According to the National Comprehensive Cancer Network (NCCN) practice guidelines, imaging at the time of staging includes chest radiography, CT or PET/CT, and MR imaging as indicated.[42] MR imaging is the preferred imaging modality to asses the extent of local disease, for delineating tumor size, endocervical margin distance, and parametrial invasion. Indeed, it has been shown that MR imaging is superior to CT for measuring tumor size.[43] However, both CT and MR imaging have limited sensitivity (31%–57% and 37%–55%, respectively) for the detection of disease spread to lymph nodes, although the specificity is reasonably good: 86% to 92% for CT and 93% to 94% for MR imaging.[44,45] PET/CT is more sensitive to evaluate disease spread to pelvic, paraaortic, and more distant lymph nodes, although the range in sensitivity is broad and decreases in early stage disease[46] or when lymph nodes are less than 5 mm.[47] In a metaanalysis of 41 studies, the sensitivity of PET/CT for the detection of lymph node disease spread was 56%, higher than MR imaging or CT alone.[48] A metaanalysis of 72 studies including 5042 women showed a pooled positive likelihood ratio of 15.3 versus 6.4 and 4.3 for the detection of lymph node disease spread using PET and PET/CT versus MR imaging versus CT, respectively.[45] The specificity of PET and PET/CT for the detection of lymph node disease spread is high, at 94% to 97%.[45,47,49,50]

Ovarian cancer

Ovarian cancer is the leading cause of gynecologic cancer death in women in the United States. It was estimated to account for 22,000 new cases and 14,000 deaths in 2016.[51] There are 2 types of epithelial ovarian cancer based on pathologic and genetic features. Type I includes low-grade serous, low-grade endometrioid, clear cell and mucinous tumors, and type II includes high-grade serous, high-grade endometrioid, and undifferentiated carcinoma.[52] Type II pathology is the most common, accounting for approximately 75% of cases and 90% of cancer-related deaths. Often diagnosed on the basis of clinical history, imaging, elevated tumor markers (CA-125), and histology, the majority of cases present with metastatic disease. The 5-year survival of cancer localized to the ovary is greater than 92%, but decreases to 29% when distant disease is present.[51]

Staging depends on findings at the time of cytoreductive surgery and biopsy according to the FIGO classification system. Prognosis depends on the extent of visible tumor resection. For patients with medical comorbidities or with a tumor burden not amenable to complete resection, treatment includes neoadjuvant chemotherapy, aggressive surgery, and additional chemotherapy. Imaging can be helpful at the time of initial evaluation and to identify patients unlikely to have resectable disease (see **Fig. 3**). MR imaging is the modality of choice for the detection of primary disease (sensitivity and specificity of 81% and 98%, respectively) and can be helpful to distinguish benign from malignant pathology.[53] According to the NCCN practice guidelines, both CT and MR imaging can be helpful to ascertain disease extent and results in the literature suggest the 2 are comparable to detect peritoneal disease spread.[54] Given accessibility and tolerability issues, CT is commonly the imaging modality of choice.

It has been shown that PET/CT can improve pretreatment staging accuracy.[55–58] A metaanalysis of 18 studies in 882 patients found PET or PET/CT had higher sensitivity and specificity to detect lymph node disease spread (73.2% and 96.7%, respectively) than CT (42.6% and 95.0%, respectively) or MR imaging (54.7% and 88.3%, respectively).[56] In particular, Nam and colleagues[57] found in their prospective study of 95 patients with ovarian cancer, PET/CT before surgical staging identified unpredicted supraabdominal lymph node disease that surgical staging did not identify in 15 cases (16%), of which 10 were supraclavicular lymph node metastases. Other studies have also shown that PET/CT is the preferred imaging modality for the detection of extraabdominal disease.[58,59] However, even though PET/CT does detect additional sites of extraabdominal disease in the preoperative setting, this may not have an effect on patient prognosis. As such, PET/CT is often not recommended for pretreatment staging.[59,60]

The ability of PET/CT to detect carcinomatosis reported in the literature is variable.[60,61] Hynninen and colleagues[60] showed that PET/CT was superior to CT for the detection of carcinomatosis on the subdiaphragmatic peritoneal surface and in the bowel mesentery, but not for the detection of carcinomatosis in other areas of the peritoneal cavity. Other researchers found multidetector CT was superior to PET/CT in the diagnosis of peritoneal seeding.[62] All in all, the American College of Radiology guidelines do not recommend PET/CT for pretreatment staging,[63] whereas the NCCN guidelines states that PET/CT may be indicated for characterizing indeterminate ovarian lesions if results will alter management.[64]

PET at Initial Diagnosis and Staging as a Biomarker of Prognosis

Prognostic value of various PET signatures in the primary lesion

The role of PET as a biomarker centers on the ability of PET to provide an early prediction of progression-free and overall survival independent of the morphologic extent of disease at diagnosis. Indeed, similar to other cancer types, the metabolic patterns of aggressive gynecologic cancer lesions can be used to stratify patients into subpopulations with different prognoses. Understanding the prognostic value of metabolism in these tumor types facilitates the identification of patients at high risk of early disease progression. This information can then be used early during the course of clinical management to personalize adjuvant and postoperative therapy in those with early stage disease, but highly metabolically active tumors.

The prognostic value of different PET signatures in gynecologic cancer has been investigated and several investigators have reported similar results in the literature. Examples of these PET signatures are the intensity of tumor metabolic activity in terms of SUV, metabolically active tumor bulk as defined by indices of metabolic volumes (MTV) and total tumor glycolysis (TLG), and tumoral metabolic heterogeneity estimated through texture analysis.

The MTV is a measure of metabolically active tumor mass and is estimated by using semiautomatic contouring software with a predefined SUV as the threshold to segment the metabolically active tumor boundaries. The TLG is calculated by multiplying the mean SUV of the tumor by the MTV. The whole body MTV and TLG can then be obtained by summing the values for each individual lesion in the body. As such, the MTV and TLG provide 3-dimensional measurements of total volume and metabolic activity associated with the cancer. High-intensity FDG uptake is associated with more aggressive gynecologic cancer and is considered a prognostic imaging biomarker in several tumor types. Indeed, the evidence suggests high tumor SUV, MTV, and TLG are associated with poor prognosis,[65–68] although not necessarily with histologic grade.[69]

The intensity of FDG uptake at the site of primary disease, MTV, and TLG are independent predictive factors for recurrence and survival in gynecologic cancer. Several studies have shown that the more intensely FDG avid the site of primary disease, the more likely the disease has spread. For example, Antonsen and colleagues[70] showed that the more intensely FDG avid the primary malignancy in women with endometrial cancer, the higher the risk of spread to lymph nodes and the more likely the patient was to have a higher FIGO stage, and myometrial and cervical invasion. Husby and colleagues[71] suggested the greater the MTV at the site of primary disease, the more likely the endometrial cancer had spread beyond the uterus. Kim and colleagues[72] found that in stage IA to IIB invasive cervical cancer, the MTV was a significant independent predictor of recurrent disease. Further, the MTV significantly differed according to tumor differentiation and patients with high MTV (>20 cm^3) had significantly decreased disease-free survival compared with patients who had a lower MTV. Micco and colleagues[73] found that the MTV and TLG were associated with high-risk features and could serve as prognostic biomarkers of survival in patients with stage IB to IVB cervical cancer. Cho and colleagues[74] and Semaan and colleagues[75] found increased GLUT-1 expression in epithelial ovarian cancer correlated with poor survival. Yamamoto and colleagues[76] showed that TLG had a 3.915-fold increase in the hazard ratio of progression-free survival in women with epithelial ovarian cancer who received platinum-based adjuvant chemotherapy after cytoreductive surgery.

Intratumoral heterogeneity may be evaluated using textural features and is considered a driver of tumor aggressiveness, resistance to treatment, and poor overall survival in several tumor types. Although there are preliminary data suggesting tumor heterogeneity based on textural features may play a role as a biomarker of prognosis in endometrial cancer,[77] the literature on the topic is sparse and there is a need for prospective, randomized trials before this can be included in daily clinical practice.

Prognostic value of ^{18}F-labeled 2-fluoro-2-deoxy-D-glucose avidity, extent of lymphadenopathy, and disease spread on PET

The intensity of FDG uptake and extent of lymph node disease spread are both prognostic markers of survival. Specifically, the more intense the disease and the more distant the lymph nodes spread, the worse the prognosis. A metaanalysis reported that the maximum SUV of paraaortic lymph nodes was associated with a pooled hazard ratio of 4.41 for death in patients with cervical cancer and was even higher than that of the combined hazard ratio of 2.45 for the maximum SUV of the primary disease.[78] Further, Kidd and colleagues[79] showed that the hazard ratio for disease recurrence increased incrementally based on the most distant level of nodal disease: pelvic 2.40, paraaortic 5.88, and supraclavicular 30.27. Similar results have been demonstrated in patients with

ovarian cancer. In particular, Caobelli and colleagues[80] showed that lymph node disease and
distant spread of ovarian cancer were independently associated with an increased risk of progression (hazard ratios of 1.6 and 2.2,
respectively). **Fig. 2** illustrates a patient with
ovarian cancer and multiple intensely FDG-avid
lymph nodes.

PET IN THE SUBSEQUENT TREATMENT STRATEGY OF GYNECOLOGIC MALIGNANCY

In gynecologic malignancy, PET is a predictive
biomarker of response to treatment. It is also a
biomarker of prognosis. As such, PET contributes
to precision medicine by influencing the decision
to treat and the type of treatment to be used.
Further, being able to detect recurrent disease
early and accurately allows clinicians to adjust
the treatment algorithm and consider second-line
therapy, as and when needed. Both PET/CT and
PET/MR imaging are superior to CT and MR imaging alone for the detection of recurrent disease
across the spectrum of gynecologic malignancy.[81]

Detection of Recurrent Disease and Restaging

Endometrial cancer
Approximately 70% to 80% of patients with endometrial cancer have disease confined to the uterus
and 10% to 20% of patients with confined disease
will develop recurrent disease within the first
3 years after initial therapy, typically those with
high-risk baseline disease.[82] Common sites of
recurrence include the vagina and lymph nodes.
Up to 20% of patients have clinically unsuspected
metastases at the time recurrent disease is
detected.[82] Bollineni and colleagues[83] suggested
the sensitivity and specificity of PET/CT for the
detection of endometrial cancer recurrence after
primary surgical treatment was high: 95% and
91%, respectively.

Cervical cancer
Approximately one-third of patients with cervical
cancer develop recurrent disease within the first
2 years after initial therapy and the presence of
recurrent disease on PET/CT is linked with survival. The sensitivity and specificity of PET/CT for
the detection of cervical cancer recurrence after
primary surgical treatment is high and the
NCCN guidelines suggest PET/CT be performed
3 to 6 months after chemoradiation has been
completed.[42] It is estimated that patients with a
negative follow-up PET/CT have a 5-year survival
of 92%, which decreases to 46% when residual
disease is present and 0% when sites of new
disease are detected.[84] **Fig. 5** shows selected

PET/CT images from a woman with localized
recurrent cervical cancer after initial treatment
with radiation and chemotherapy and a complete
response to additional chemotherapy. The PET/
CT was particularly helpful in that it (1) pinpointed
the metabolically active recurrent cervical cancer,
(2) clarified an equivocal finding in the left femoral
head on MR imaging, and (3) showed the complete
anatomic and metabolic response to additional
chemotherapy.

Ovarian cancer
Approximately 75% of patients with ovarian cancer relapse, despite initial response to therapy,
and almost all of the patients who relapse die
from their disease.[85] Surveillance includes phys-
ical examination and serial serum CA-125 measurements with imaging reserved for those in
whom recurrence is clinically suspected. PET/CT
has been shown to have better diagnostic performance than CT or MR imaging for the evaluation
of recurrent disease. In a metaanalysis of 34
studies, Gu and colleagues[86] found the pooled
sensitivity and specificity for the detection of
recurrent ovarian cancer was 79% and 84%,
respectively, for CT, 75% and 78%, respectively,
for MR imaging, and 91% and 88%, respectively,
for PET/CT.

PET/CT has also been shown to alter management in as many as 44% to 60% of patients,
although the impact of PET/CT on patient management varies across studies in the literature.[87–89] Also, the impact seems to vary
depending on clinical setting. For example, Han
and colleagues[90] found PET/CT, when performed
for surveillance, changed management in approximately 11% of cases, whereas PET/CT excluded
disease recurrence in 17% of patients with clinical
suspicion.

Midtherapy and Posttherapy PET for Monitoring Treatment Response and as a Predictive Biomarker of Outcome

Metabolic imaging with PET as a predictive
biomarker of gynecologic cancer response to therapy is based in part on the fact that metabolic and
pathophysiologic changes often precede
anatomic change. Indeed, PET tends to predict
response to treatment earlier than imaging modalities that focus on anatomic change (ie, CT and MR
imaging). Martoni and colleagues[91] found that, in
42 patients with ovarian cancer on neoadjuvant
carboplatin-paclitaxel chemotherapy, those with
metabolically active disease after 3 cycles were
likely to benefit from surgical excision of refractory
disease before additional chemotherapy. Those
patients with a complete metabolic response on

PET/CT after 3 cycles, were likely to have complete pathologic response or minimal residual disease after 6 cycles of chemotherapy. Vallius and colleagues[92] also showed that a metabolic response on PET/CT was associated with a histopathologic response in patients with ovarian cancer. The literature suggests the earlier and more significant the response of the metabolically active malignant gynecologic disease to therapy, the longer the survival of the cancer patient (see **Fig. 5**), whereas patients who do not show a metabolic response to therapy have lower overall survival (see **Fig. 4**).[80,93] Indeed, a metaanalysis of 1854 patients from 16 studies showed a statistically significant association between pretreatment PET or PET/CT, metabolic response to therapy, and overall survival.[94]

SUMMARY

PET (either as PET/CT or PET/MR imaging) is an important molecular imaging technique with a major role in the precision medicine algorithm of patients with gynecologic malignancy. These hybrid imaging modalities provide anatomofunctional insight during diagnosis, staging, and restaging. However, they can be used as a biomarker of disease aggressiveness and heterogeneity that directs the selection of the most appropriate treatment, and predicts response early and accurately during the course of therapy.

REFERENCES

1. Cotran RS, Kumar V, Collins T. Robbins pathologic basis of disease. 6th edition. Saunders; 1999. p. 1035–93.
2. Lee SI, Catalano OA, Dehdashti F. Evaluation of gynecologic cancer with MR imaging, 18F-FDG PET/CT, and PET/MR imaging. J Nucl Med 2015;56:436–43.
3. Sharma SK, Nemieboka B, Sala E, et al. Molecular imaging of ovarian cancer. J Nucl Med 2016;57: 827–33.
4. Faubion SS, MacLaughlin KL, Long ME, et al. Surveillance and care of the gynecologic cancer survivor. J Womens Health (Larchmt) 2015;24:899–906.
5. Nogami Y, Iida M, Banno K, et al. Application of FDG-PET in cervical cancer and endometrial cancer: utility and future prospects. Anticancer Res 2014;34:585–92.
6. Prabhakar HB, Kraeft JJ, Schorge JO, et al. FDG PET-CT of gynecologic cancers: pearls and pitfalls. Abdom Imaging 2015;40:2472–85.
7. Hillner BE, Siegel BA, Shields AF, et al. Relationship between cancer type and impact of PET and PET/CT on intended management: findings of the national oncologic PET registry. J Nucl Med 2008;49:1928–35.
8. Scheuermann JS, Saffer JR, Karp JS, et al. Qualification of PET scanners for use in multicenter cancer clinical trials: the American College of Radiology Imaging Network experience. J Nucl Med 2009;50: 1187–93.
9. Boellaard R, Rausch I, Beyer T, et al. Quality control for quantitative multicenter whole-body PET/MR studies: a NEMA image quality phantom study with three current PET/MR systems. Med Phys 2015;42:5961–9.
10. Drzezga A, Souvatzoglou M, Eiber M, et al. First clinical experience with integrated whole-body PET/MR: comparison to PET/CT in patients with oncologic diagnoses. J Nucl Med 2012;53:845–55.
11. Rauscher I, Eiber M, Furst S, et al. PET/MR imaging in the detection and characterization of pulmonary lesions: technical and diagnostic evaluation in comparison to PET/CT. J Nucl Med 2014;55:724–9.
12. Richard SD, Bencherif B, Edwards RP, et al. Noninvasive assessment of cell proliferation in ovarian cancer using [18F] 3'deoxy-3-fluorothymidine positron emission tomography/computed tomography imaging. Nucl Med Biol 2011;38:485–91.
13. Cho LP, Kim CK, Viswanathan AN. Pilot study assessing (18)F-fluorothymidine PET/CT in cervical and vaginal cancers before and after external beam radiation. Gynecol Oncol Rep 2015;14:34–7.
14. Dehdashti F, Grigsby PW, Lewis JS, et al. Assessing tumor hypoxia in cervical cancer by PET with 60Cu-labeled diacetyl-bis(N4-methylthiosemicarbazone). J Nucl Med 2008;49:201–5.
15. Tsujikawa T, Yoshida Y, Kudo T, et al. Functional images reflect aggressiveness of endometrial carcinoma: estrogen receptor expression combined with 18F-FDG PET. J Nucl Med 2009;50:1598–604.
16. Dehdashti F, Grigsby PW, Mintun MA, et al. Assessing tumor hypoxia in cervical cancer by positron emission tomography with 60Cu-ATSM: relationship to therapeutic response-a preliminary report. Int J Radiat Oncol Biol Phys 2003;55:1233–8.
17. Pecorelli S. Revised FIGO staging for carcinoma of the vulva, cervix, and endometrium. Int J Gynaecol Obstet 2009;105:103–4.
18. Hirschowitz L, Nucci M, Zaino RJ. Problematic issues in the staging of endometrial, cervical and vulval carcinomas. Histopathology 2013;62:176–202.
19. Saida T, Tanaka YO, Matsumoto K, et al. Revised FIGO staging system for cancer of the ovary, fallopian tube, and peritoneum: important implications for radiologists. Jpn J Radiol 2016;34:117–24.
20. American Joint Committee on Cancer. AJCC cancer staging manual. 7th edition. Springer; 2010. p. 395–428.
21. Micco M, Sala E, Lakhman Y, et al. Role of imaging in the pretreatment evaluation of common gynecological cancers. Womens Health (Lond) 2014;10:299–321.
22. Queiroz MA, Kubik-Huch RA, Hauser N, et al. PET/MRI and PET/CT in advanced gynaecological

tumours: initial experience and comparison. Eur Radiol 2015;25:2222–30.

23. National Cancer Institute. Cancer stat facts: endometrial cancer. Available at: https://seer.cancer.gov/statfacts/html/corp.html. Accessed March 9, 2017.

24. Bokhman JV. Two pathogenetic types of endometrial carcinoma. Gynecol Oncol 1983;15:10–7.

25. Evans T, Sany O, Pearmain P, et al. Differential trends in the rising incidence of endometrial cancer by type: data from a UK population-based registry from 1994 to 2006. Br J Cancer 2011;104:1505–10.

26. Tanaka K, Kobayashi Y, Sugiyama J, et al. Histologic grade and peritoneal cytology as prognostic factors in type 1 endometrial cancer. Int J Clin Oncol 2017;22(3):533–40.

27. Creasman WT, Morrow CP, Bundy BN, et al. Surgical pathologic spread patterns of endometrial cancer. A Gynecologic Oncology Group Study. Cancer 1987;60:2035–41.

28. Creasman WT, DeGeest K, DiSaia PJ, et al. Significance of true surgical pathologic staging: a Gynecologic Oncology Group Study. Am J Obstet Gynecol 1999;181:31–4.

29. Lewin SN, Herzog TJ, Barrena Medel NI, et al. Comparative performance of the 2009 International Federation of Gynecology and Obstetrics' staging system for uterine corpus cancer. Obstet Gynecol 2010;116:1141–9.

30. Mariani A, Dowdy SC, Cliby WA, et al. Prospective assessment of lymphatic dissemination in endometrial cancer: a paradigm shift in surgical staging. Gynecol Oncol 2008;109:11–8.

31. Rossi EC, Kowalski LD, Scalici J, et al. A comparison of sentinel lymph node biopsy to lymphadenectomy for endometrial cancer staging (FIRES trial): a multicentre, prospective, cohort study. Lancet Oncol 2017;18:384–92.

32. Koh WJ, Greer BE, Abu-Rustum NR, et al. Uterine neoplasms, version 1.2014. J Natl Compr Canc Netw 2014;12:248–80.

33. Duncan KA, Drinkwater KJ, Frost C, et al. Staging cancer of the uterus: a national audit of MRI accuracy. Clin Radiol 2012;67:523–30.

34. Antonsen SL, Jensen LN, Loft A, et al. MRI, PET/CT and ultrasound in the preoperative staging of endometrial cancer - a multicenter prospective comparative study. Gynecol Oncol 2013;128:300–8.

35. Signorelli M, Guerra L, Buda A, et al. Role of the integrated FDG PET/CT in the surgical management of patients with high risk clinical early stage endometrial cancer: detection of pelvic nodal metastases. Gynecol Oncol 2009;115:231–5.

36. Selman TJ, Mann CH, Zamora J, et al. A systematic review of tests for lymph node status in primary endometrial cancer. BMC Womens Health 2008;8:8.

37. Picchio M, Mangili G, Samanes Gajate AM, et al. High-grade endometrial cancer: value of [(18)F] FDG PET/CT in preoperative staging. Nucl Med Commun 2010;31:506–12.

38. Sironi S, Picchio M, Landoni C, et al. Post-therapy surveillance of patients with uterine cancers: value of integrated FDG PET/CT in the detection of recurrence. Eur J Nucl Med Mol Imaging 2007;34:472–9.

39. Kitajima K, Murakami K, Yamasaki E, et al. Performance of FDG-PET/CT in the diagnosis of recurrent endometrial cancer. Ann Nucl Med 2008;22:103–9.

40. Atri M, Zhang Z, Dehdashti F, et al. Utility of PET/CT to evaluate retroperitoneal lymph node metastasis in high-risk endometrial cancer: results of ACRIN 6671/GOG 0233 trial. Radiology 2017;283(2):450–9.

41. National Cancer Institute. Cancer stat facts: cervix uteri cancer. Available at: https://seer.cancer.gov/statfacts/html/cervix.html. Accessed March 9, 2017.

42. Koh WJ, Greer BE, Abu-Rustum NR, et al. Cervical cancer. J Natl Compr Canc Netw 2013;11:320–43.

43. Mitchell DG, Snyder B, Coakley F, et al. Early invasive cervical cancer: tumor delineation by magnetic resonance imaging, computed tomography, and clinical examination, verified by pathologic results, in the ACRIN 6651/GOG 183 Intergroup Study. J Clin Oncol 2006;24:5687–94.

44. Hricak H, Gatsonis C, Chi DS, et al. Role of imaging in pretreatment evaluation of early invasive cervical cancer: results of the intergroup study American College of Radiology Imaging Network 6651-Gynecologic Oncology Group 183. J Clin Oncol 2005;23:9329–37.

45. Selman TJ, Mann C, Zamora J, et al. Diagnostic accuracy of tests for lymph node status in primary cervical cancer: a systematic review and meta-analysis. CMAJ 2008;178:855–62.

46. Signorelli M, Guerra L, Montanelli L, et al. Preoperative staging of cervical cancer: is 18-FDG-PET/CT really effective in patients with early stage disease? Gynecol Oncol 2011;123:236–40.

47. Roh JW, Seo SS, Lee S, et al. Role of positron emission tomography in pretreatment lymph node staging of uterine cervical cancer: a prospective surgicopathologic correlation study. Eur J Cancer 2005;41:2086–92.

48. Choi HJ, Ju W, Myung SK, et al. Diagnostic performance of computer tomography, magnetic resonance imaging, and positron emission tomography or positron emission tomography/computer tomography for detection of metastatic lymph nodes in patients with cervical cancer: meta-analysis. Cancer Sci 2010;101:1471–9.

49. Loft A, Berthelsen AK, Roed H, et al. The diagnostic value of PET/CT scanning in patients with cervical cancer: a prospective study. Gynecol Oncol 2007;106:29–34.

50. Lin WC, Hung YC, Yeh LS, et al. Usefulness of (18) F-fluorodeoxyglucose positron emission tomography to detect para-aortic lymph nodal metastasis in advanced cervical cancer with negative computed tomography findings. Gynecol Oncol 2003;89:73–6.

51. National Cancer Institute. Cancer stat facts: ovarian cancer. Available at: https://seer.cancer.gov/statfacts/html/ovary.html. Accessed March 9, 2017.

52. Kurman RJ, Shih Ie M. The origin and pathogenesis of epithelial ovarian cancer: a proposed unifying theory. Am J Surg Pathol 2010;34:433–43.

53. Kinkel K, Lu Y, Mehdizade A, et al. Indeterminate ovarian mass at US: incremental value of second imaging test for characterization–meta-analysis and Bayesian analysis. Radiology 2005;236:85–94.

54. National Comprehensive Cancer Network. NCCN National Guidelines for patients – Ovarian caner. Available at: https://www.nccn.org/patients/guidelines/ovarian/index.html#18. Accessed March 10, 2017.

55. Castellucci P, Perrone AM, Picchio M, et al. Diagnostic accuracy of 18F-FDG PET/CT in characterizing ovarian lesions and staging ovarian cancer: correlation with transvaginal ultrasonography, computed tomography, and histology. Nucl Med Commun 2007;28:589–95.

56. Yuan Y, Gu ZX, Tao XF, et al. Computer tomography, magnetic resonance imaging, and positron emission tomography or positron emission tomography/computer tomography for detection of metastatic lymph nodes in patients with ovarian cancer: a meta-analysis. Eur J Radiol 2012;81:1002–6.

57. Nam EJ, Yun MJ, Oh YT, et al. Diagnosis and staging of primary ovarian cancer: correlation between PET/CT, Doppler US, and CT or MRI. Gynecol Oncol 2010;116:389–94.

58. Risum S, Hogdall C, Loft A, et al. Does the use of diagnostic PET/CT cause stage migration in patients with primary advanced ovarian cancer? Gynecol Oncol 2010;116:395–8.

59. Fruscio R, Sina F, Dolci C, et al. Preoperative 18F-FDG PET/CT in the management of advanced epithelial ovarian cancer. Gynecol Oncol 2013;131:689–93.

60. Hynninen J, Kemppainen J, Lavonius M, et al. A prospective comparison of integrated FDG-PET/contrast-enhanced CT and contrast-enhanced CT for pretreatment imaging of advanced epithelial ovarian cancer. Gynecol Oncol 2013;131:389–94.

61. Schmidt S, Meuli RA, Achtari C, et al. Peritoneal carcinomatosis in primary ovarian cancer staging: comparison between MDCT, MRI, and 18F-FDG PET/CT. Clin Nucl Med 2015;40:371–7.

62. Funicelli L, Travaini LL, Landoni F, et al. Peritoneal carcinomatosis from ovarian cancer: the role of CT and [(1)(8)F]FDG-PET/CT. Abdom Imaging 2010;35:701–7.

63. Mitchell DG, Javitt MC, Glanc P, et al. ACR appropriateness criteria staging and follow-up of ovarian cancer. J Am Coll Radiol 2013;10:822–7.

64. NCCN clinical practice guidelines in oncology: Ovarian cancer including fallopian tube cancer and primary peritoneal cancer. Version 1. 2016. Available at: http://www.nccn.org/professionals/physician_gls/pdf/ovarian.pdf. Accessed March 15, 2017.

65. Kidd EA, Siegel BA, Dehdashti F, et al. The standardized uptake value for F-18 fluorodeoxyglucose is a sensitive predictive biomarker for cervical cancer treatment response and survival. Cancer 2007;110:1738–44.

66. Chung HH, Kwon HW, Kang KW, et al. Prognostic value of preoperative metabolic tumor volume and total lesion glycolysis in patients with epithelial ovarian cancer. Ann Surg Oncol 2012;19:1966–72.

67. Chung HH, Lee I, Kim HS, et al. Prognostic value of preoperative metabolic tumor volume measured by (1)(8)F-FDG PET/CT and MRI in patients with endometrial cancer. Gynecol Oncol 2013;130:446–51.

68. Shim SH, Kim DY, Lee DY, et al. Metabolic tumour volume and total lesion glycolysis, measured using preoperative 18F-FDG PET/CT, predict the recurrence of endometrial cancer. BJOG 2014;121:1097–106 [discussion: 1106].

69. Mocciaro V, Scollo P, Stefano A, et al. Correlation between histological grade and positron emission tomography parameters in cervical carcinoma. Oncol Lett 2016;12:1408–14.

70. Antonsen SL, Loft A, Fisker R, et al. SUVmax of 18FDG PET/CT as a predictor of high-risk endometrial cancer patients. Gynecol Oncol 2013;129:298–303.

71. Husby JA, Reitan BC, Biermann M, et al. Metabolic tumor volume on 18F-FDG PET/CT improves preoperative identification of high-risk endometrial carcinoma patients. J Nucl Med 2015;56:1191–8.

72. Kim BS, Kim IJ, Kim SJ, et al. The prognostic value of the metabolic tumor volume in FIGO stage IA to IIB cervical cancer for tumor recurrence: measured by F-18 FDG PET/CT. Nucl Med Mol Imaging 2011;45:36–42.

73. Micco M, Vargas HA, Burger IA, et al. Combined pre-treatment MRI and 18F-FDG PET/CT parameters as prognostic biomarkers in patients with cervical cancer. Eur J Radiol 2014;83:1169–76.

74. Cho H, Lee YS, Kim J, et al. Overexpression of glucose transporter-1 (GLUT-1) predicts poor prognosis in epithelial ovarian cancer. Cancer Invest 2013;31:607–15.

75. Semaan A, Munkarah AR, Arabi H, et al. Expression of GLUT-1 in epithelial ovarian carcinoma: correlation with tumor cell proliferation, angiogenesis, survival and ability to predict optimal cytoreduction. Gynecol Oncol 2011;121:181–6.

76. Yamamoto M, Tsujikawa T, Fujita Y, et al. Metabolic tumor burden predicts prognosis of ovarian cancer patients who receive platinum-based adjuvant chemotherapy. Cancer Sci 2016;107:478–85.

77. Kang SY, Cheon GJ, Lee M, et al. Prediction of recurrence by preoperative intratumoral FDG uptake heterogeneity in endometrioid endometrial cancer. Transl Oncol 2017;10:178–83.

78. Sarker A, Im HJ, Cheon GJ, et al. Prognostic implications of the SUVmax of primary tumors and metastatic lymph node measured by 18F-FDG PET in patients with uterine cervical cancer: a meta-analysis. Clin Nucl Med 2016;41:34–40.

79. Kidd EA, Siegel BA, Dehdashti F, et al. Lymph node staging by positron emission tomography in cervical cancer: relationship to prognosis. J Clin Oncol 2010; 28:2108–13.

80. Caobelli F, Alongi P, Evangelista L, et al. Predictive value of (18)F-FDG PET/CT in restaging patients affected by ovarian carcinoma: a multicentre study. Eur J Nucl Med Mol Imaging 2016;43:404–13.

81. Kirchner J, Sawicki LM, Suntharalingam S, et al. Whole-body staging of female patients with recurrent pelvic malignancies: ultra-fast 18F-FDG PET/ MRI compared to 18F-FDG PET/CT and CT. PLoS One 2017;12:e0172553.

82. Berchuck A, Anspach C, Evans AC, et al. Postsurgical surveillance of patients with FIGO stage I/II endometrial adenocarcinoma. Gynecol Oncol 1995;59:20–4.

83. Bollineni VR, Ytre-Hauge S, Bollineni-Balabay O, et al. High diagnostic value of 18F-FDG PET/CT in endometrial cancer: systematic review and meta-analysis of the literature. J Nucl Med 2016;57: 879–85.

84. Grigsby PW, Siegel BA, Dehdashti F, et al. Posttherapy [18F] fluorodeoxyglucose positron emission tomography in carcinoma of the cervix: response and outcome. J Clin Oncol 2004;22:2167–71.

85. Gadducci A, Cosio S, Zola P, et al. Surveillance procedures for patients treated for epithelial ovarian cancer: a review of the literature. Int J Gynecol Cancer 2007;17:21–31.

86. Gu P, Pan LL, Wu SQ, et al. CA 125, PET alone, PET-CT, CT and MRI in diagnosing recurrent ovarian carcinoma: a systematic review and meta-analysis. Eur J Radiol 2009;71:164–74.

87. Mangili G, Picchio M, Sironi S, et al. Integrated PET/ CT as a first-line re-staging modality in patients with suspected recurrence of ovarian cancer. Eur J Nucl Med Mol Imaging 2007;34:658–66.

88. Simcock B, Neesham D, Quinn M, et al. The impact of PET/CT in the management of recurrent ovarian cancer. Gynecol Oncol 2006;103:271–6.

89. Fulham MJ, Carter J, Baldey A, et al. The impact of PET-CT in suspected recurrent ovarian cancer: a prospective multi-centre study as part of the Australian PET Data Collection Project. Gynecol Oncol 2009;112:462–8.

90. Han EJ, Park HL, Lee YS, et al. Clinical usefulness of post-treatment FDG PET/CT in patients with ovarian malignancy. Ann Nucl Med 2016;30:600–7.

91. Martoni AA, Fanti S, Zamagni C, et al. [18F]FDG-PET/CT monitoring early identifies advanced ovarian cancer patients who will benefit from prolonged neoadjuvant chemotherapy. Q J Nucl Med Mol Imaging 2011;55:81–90.

92. Vallius T, Peter A, Auranen A, et al. 18F-FDG-PET/CT can identify histopathological non-responders to platinum-based neoadjuvant chemotherapy in advanced epithelial ovarian cancer. Gynecol Oncol 2016;140:29–35.

93. Tanaka Y, Ueda Y, Egawa-Takata T, et al. Early metabolic change in (18)F-FDG-PET by measuring the single largest lesion predicts chemotherapeutic effects and patients' survival: PEACH study. Cancer Chemother Pharmacol 2016;77:121–6.

94. Zhao Q, Feng Y, Mao X, et al. Prognostic value of fluorine-18-fluorodeoxyglucose positron emission tomography or PET-computed tomography in cervical cancer: a meta-analysis. Int J Gynecol Cancer 2013; 23:1184–90.

PET–Computed Tomography and Precision Medicine in Pancreatic Adenocarcinoma and Pancreatic Neuroendocrine Tumors

Daniella F. Pinho, MD[a],*,
Rathan M. Subramaniam, MD, PhD, MPH[a,b,c,d,e]

KEYWORDS

- Pancreatic cancer • Pancreatic adenocarcinoma • Pancreatic neuroendocrine tumor • PET
- PET/CT

KEY POINTS

- ^{18}F-fluorodeoxyglucose (FDG) PET/computed tomography (CT) has good sensitivity and specificity for diagnosis of pancreatic adenocarcinoma. It has also shown benefit for detection of local and distant metastatic disease.
- Evaluation of response to treatment has shown good rate of recurrence detection by FDG PET/CT, especially in patients undergoing surgery. Pretreatment FDG PET/CT volume-based parameters can reliably predict a patient's outcome.
- Fluorothymidine (FLT) is a more recent PET tracer that evaluates tumor proliferation and has the potential to be more specific than FDG PET/CT, especially on the evaluation of response to treatment.
- ^{68}Ga-DOTA-labeled somatostatin analogues are superior for detection of well-differentiated neuroendocrine tumors compared with conventional imaging modalities.
- The NETTER-1 trial has shown survival benefit with treatment using 177-lutetium DOTATATE in patients with metastatic neuroendocrine tumors compared with high-dose octreotide treatment.

Pancreatic adenocarcinoma has a very poor prognosis as patients are usually diagnosed with locally advanced or metastatic disease and current therapies are not efficient to increase patient's survival. A multimodality approach is currently used for diagnosis, staging and evaluation of recurrence, including computed tomography, magnetic resonance, endoscopic ultrasound and FDG PET/CT, with different strengths for each modality. ^{18}F-FDG PET/CT has been described as an accurate

[a] Department of Radiology, The University of Texas Southwestern Medical Center, 5323 Harry Hines Boulevard, Dallas, TX 75390-8896, USA; [b] Department of Clinical Sciences, The University of Texas Southwestern Medical Center, 5323 Harry Hines Boulevard, Dallas, TX 75390-8896, USA; [c] Department of Biomedical Engineering, The University of Texas Southwestern Medical Center, 5323 Harry Hines Boulevard, Dallas, TX 75390-8896, USA; [d] Advanced Imaging Research Center, The University of Texas Southwestern Medical Center, 5323 Harry Hines Boulevard, Dallas, TX 75390-8896, USA; [e] Harold C. Simmons Comprehensive Cancer Center, The University of Texas Southwestern Medical Center, 5323 Harry Hines Boulevard, Dallas, TX 75390-8896, USA
* Corresponding author.
E-mail address: Daniella.Pinho@UTSouthwestern.edu

PET Clin 12 (2017) 407–421
http://dx.doi.org/10.1016/j.cpet.2017.05.003
1556-8598/17/© 2017 Elsevier Inc. All rights reserved.

tool for initial diagnosis of pancreatic adenocarcinoma, by differentiating benign from malignant etiologies, useful for metastatic disease detection including local lymphadenopathy and especially for distant spread of disease. More recent studies showed that ^{18}F-FDG PET/CT is also a very good predictor of patient prognosis. Its role to evaluate response to surgery and chemoradiation is also evolving. ^{18}F-FLT is a new PET tracer that has the potential to be more specific for tumor proliferation. Lately, textural analysis of PET has shown promising results to predict patient's outcome.

Pancreatic neuroendocrine tumors (NETs) are rare tumors that originate from the islet cells of the pancreas. NETs are predominantly well-differentiated tumors that are usually nonfunctional but can be associated with hormonal syndromes. Imaging of the pancreatic NET targets the somatostatin receptors (SSTRs) that are overexpressed in its surface by using SSTR analogues, such as ^{111}In-diethylenetriaminepentacetic acid (DTPA)-octreotide for gamma camera and single-proton emission computed tomography (SPECT)–computed tomography (CT) imaging, and of ^{68}Ga-DOTA (1,4,7,10-tetraazacyclododecane-1,4,7,10-tetraacetic acid)-labeled somatostatin analogues for PET/CT imaging. Currently, ^{68}Ga-DOTA-labeled somatostatin analogues are considered the best modality for detection of NETs. ^{18}F-fluorodeoxyglucose (FDG) PET/CT has a role in patients with poorly differentiated tumors. Recent studies have demonstrated improved survival in patients with metastatic NETs treated with 90-yttrium (Y) and 177-lutetium (Lu) as radionuclides compared with treatment with octreotide.

PANCREATIC DUCTAL ADENOCARCINOMA
Introduction

Pancreatic ductal adenocarcinoma (PDAC) is the fourth most lethal malignancy overall, with a projected death toll of more than 600,000 for 2016 in the United States.[1] Pancreatic adenocarcinoma is usually locally advanced and/or metastatic at the time of diagnosis, preventing surgical resection in most cases. Multiagent chemotherapy regimens are usually used in patients who are not candidates for resection, including leucovorin plus fluorouracil (FU), oxaliplatin and irinotecan (FOLFIRINOX) or gemcitabine plus nanoparticle albumin-bound paclitaxel (nab-paclitaxel), which are associated with significantly prolonged survival compared with gemcitabine alone.[2–5] Understanding the unique characteristics of each tumor may lead to personalized medicine, with potential for early detection, specific targeted therapies, and prognostic prediction in these patients.

Molecular Genetics

Elucidation of molecular mechanisms provides insights in understanding the progression of normal pancreatic ductal cells to noninvasive precursor lesions and to invasive carcinoma. Genome sequencing analysis of PDAC revealed an average of 119 somatic chromosomal structural variants per individual patient.[6] The mutations were related to 12 different core signaling pathways, altered in 67% to 100% of the tumors.

The most common categories for mutations found in patients with pancreatic adenocarcinoma were mutational activation of oncogenes (kirsten rat sarcoma viral oncogene homolog [K-Ras]), inactivation of tumor suppressor genes (ie, tumor protein p53, p16/cyclin-dependent kinase inhibitor 2A [CDKN2A] and SMAD family member 4 [SMAD4]), and inactivation of genome maintenance genes, which control the repair of DNA damage (ie, hMLH1 and MSH2). K-Ras mutations are often the initiating event, followed by the 3 tumor suppressor genes (TP53, p16/CDKN2A, and SMAD4).[7–9]

Although there are many different genetic mutations found on PDAC, most are involved in a few common signaling pathways (Fig. 1). See later discussion of some of the most important signaling pathways in pancreatic cancer and their role in personalized medicine. Because most of the attempts of direct therapy to pancreatic adenocarcinoma haven not yet shown relevant clinical benefit, imaging studies to assess response to treatment with molecular target therapies lack in the literature.

Epidermal growth factor receptor signaling
Multiple growth factors and their ligands are overexpressed in PDACs. Epidermal growth factor (EGF) and transforming growth factor alpha (TGF-a) activate EGF receptor (EGFR), a transmembrane tyrosine kinase receptor. It is detected in 90% of PDACs and plays a role in liver metastasis and recurrence of tumor.[10] Overexpression of EGFR is also seen in a variety of solid tumors, including prostate, breast, colon, and non-small cell lung cancer.[11–13] Approaches targeting EGFR include monoclonal antibodies directed against the extracellular domain of the receptor (eg, cetuximab) and small molecule tyrosine kinase inhibitors of EGFR (eg, erlotinib).[14]

A large phase III study that enrolled 745 subjects compared gemcitabine alone with a combination of gemcitabine and cetuximab did not show any benefit in terms of response rate or survival with

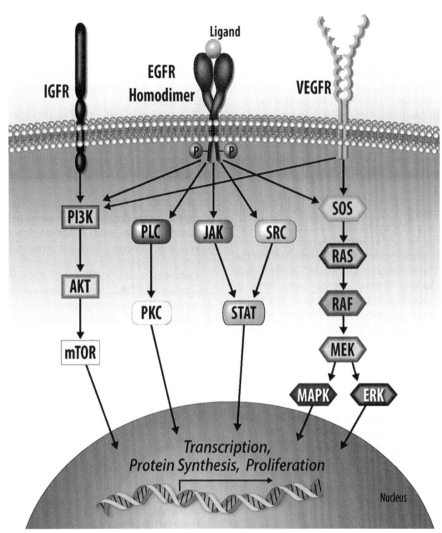

Fig. 1. Simplified representation of oncogenic signaling cascades in pancreatic cancer. Binding of ligands to receptors for IGF, EGFR, and VEGF activates downstream targets such as mTOR, PKC, STAT and MAPK, which target the nucleus for transcription, protein synthesis, and proliferation. EGFR, epidermal growth factor receptor; IGF, insulin-like growth factor; MAPK, mitogen activated protein kinase; mTOR, mechanistic target of rapamycin; PKC, protein kinase C; STAT, signal transducer and activator of transcription; VEGF, vascular endothelial growth factor.

the addition of the monoclonal antibody to the therapeutic regimen.[15] Investigators suggested that the complex signaling pathways with crosstalk prevent effective blockade of proliferative and antiapoptotic signals in advanced pancreatic, urging the need of multitargeted strategies for effectiveness.

A phase III trial compared gemcitabine alone and associated with erlotinib in 569 subjects with locally advanced or metastatic pancreatic cancer, and showed that combined therapy was better and associated with significant, although small, increase in overall survival (OS) when combined with single-therapy gemcitabine (6.2 vs 5.9 months, respectively).[16]

Vascular endothelial growth factor signaling
A continuous supply of oxygen and nutrients is needed for tumors to keep their malignant growth. Pancreatic cancer has increased expression of vascular endothelial growth factor (VEGF), which induces angiogenesis and lymphangiogenesis.[17,18] There are also 2 class III transmembrane protein tyrosine kinases cognate receptors (flk-1/KDR and flt-1), which bind VEGF with high affinity.[19] Flt-1 expression is increased in ischemia and inflammation, and upregulated in many types of tumors, in which it is associated with poor prognosis, metastasis, and recurrence.[20]

Bevacizumab is a monoclonal antibody that targets the VEGF and, although preliminary studies have shown promising results,[21] a phase III trial showed no benefit in the association of gemcitabine with bevacizumab compared with gemcitabine alone in 602 subjects with advanced pancreatic cancer.[22] Another trial compared the addition of bevacizumab to a combination of gemcitabine plus erlotinib compared with the same combination without bevacizumab and showed significant but small improvement of progression-free survival (PFS) (4.6 vs 3.6 months) but no difference in OS.[23]

K-Ras signaling

The K-Ras is an oncogene located on chromosome 12p and one of the most frequently mutated gene in pancreatic cancer, present in more than 90% of the cases.[7,24] The mutation is present in the low-grade precursor lesions (PanIn), hence very early in pancreatic carcinogenesis. This makes this oncogene an attractive target development of early detection molecular imaging. K-Ras activation is necessary for initiation, as well as for maintenance, of pancreatic cancer cells.[25] Ras proteins are part of the small G protein superfamily, and are regulated by guanine nucleotides like GTP (activation) and GDP (inactivation). Attempts to target K-Ras for the treatment of advanced pancreatic cancer have been applied to different stages of the RAS molecular pathway, with promising preclinical (stage I) results, but no clinical benefits showed yet.[26]

^{18}F-Fluorodeoxyglucose PET–Computed Tomography in Diagnosis and Staging of Pancreatic Adenocarcinoma

Preoperative diagnosis of PDAC remains a challenge in some cases, even with a multimodality approach that includes ultrasound (US), endoscopic US, CT and/or MR imaging.[27]

Differentiation between benign and malignant processes is important to guide initial evaluation and treatment of these patients. Additionally, assessment of local resectability and distant metastasis is key for determining treatment options when considering chemotherapy and surgical resection.

The usefulness of ^{18}F-FDG PET/CT for the differentiation of pancreatic adenocarcinoma from other benign conditions, such as benign biliary strictures and focal pancreatitis, has been reported by different studies[27–34] with the sensitivity ranging from 85% to 97% and the specificity from 64% to 94% for the primary tumor (Table 1). Also, increased sensitivity for detection of pancreatic adenocarcinoma was reported when using a contrast-enhanced CT when compared with unenhanced CT on the PET/CT studies.[30]

Limitations of ^{18}F-FDG PET/CT on the initial diagnosis of PDAC include false-negative studies in patients with hyperglycemia[35] and small tumors (T1 or T2),[28,36,37] as well as false-positive results related to inflammatory changes (acute, chronic, and autoimmune pancreatitis), which were shown to have increased FDG uptake, resulting in decreased specificity.[38–40]

Using FDG-PET for detection of local spread of PDAC has not shown advantages compared with local staging by conventional CT, related to the lack of detailed anatomic information given by PET/CT.[35,41] Spread of tumor to local lymph nodes is not optimally studied with CT because a size criteria (>1 cm in the short axis) cannot reliably differentiate benign, reactive lymph nodes from malignancy involvement.[42] ^{18}F-FDG PET/CT has a reported slightly better performance for lymph node detection in patients with pancreatic adenocarcinoma with a sensitivity ranging from 30% to 53%, higher when compared with conventional CT[27,43] (Fig. 2).

Table 1
Studies in diagnosis of primary pancreatic adenocarcinoma using ^{18}F-fluorodeoxyglucose PET–computed tomography

Study	Number of Subjects	Sensitivity (%)	Specificity (%)	PPV (%)	NPV (%)
Rose et al,[34] 1999	81	92	85	96	73
Lemke et al,[31] 2004	104	89	64	81	76
Heinrich et al,[28] 2005	59	89	69	91	64
Bang et al,[60] 2006	102	97	78	98	70
Schick et al,[29] 2008	46	89	74	83	82
Kauhanen et al,[27] 2009	38	85	94	94	85
Buchs et al,[30] 2011	45	96	67	92	80
Santhosh et al,[33] 2013	87	93	90	95	87

Abbreviations: NPV, negative predictive value; PPV, positive predictive value.

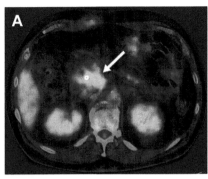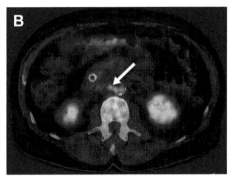

Fig. 2. ^{18}F-FDG PET/CT images of a 61-year-old man with pancreatic adenocarcinoma of the head of the pancreas (*arrow*) seen on fused PET/CT image (*A*). Additional FDG avid lymph node is seen in the aortocaval region (*arrow*), consistent with site of metastatic disease (*B*).

Detection of additional sites of distant metastatic disease in patients with PDAC is important because it prevents unnecessary resection in patients previously classified as resectable by conventional anatomic imaging. Controversial studies have been reported on the added value of ^{18}F-FDG PET/CT for diagnosis of distant metastatic disease. Kim and colleagues[44] evaluated the role of ^{18}F-FDG PET/CT for the detection of distant metastasis of PDAC. A total of 125 subjects with pretreatment ^{18}F-FDG PET/CT were included in the study. Of the 76 subjects that were determined to have resectable disease by conventional workup, only 2 had additional metastatic disease detected by ^{18}F-FDG PET/CT. The study concluded that FDG PET/CT has a limited role in the evaluation of metastatic disease from PDAC.

However, other studies have shown benefit of using ^{18}F-FDG PET/CT for detection of distant metastatic disease. Heinrich and colleagues[28] reported detection of distant metastatic disease in 5 of 59 subjects, significantly affecting management in 16% of the subjects. Additionally, Diederichs and colleagues[35] reported ^{18}F-FDG PET/CT sensitivity of 70% to detect hepatic metastasis, which increased to 93% when considering lesions greater than 1 cm. Asagi and colleagues[45] reported sensitivity of 94%. Chang and colleagues[46] studied a large population of 388 subjects and found unsuspected distant metastasis in 33% of the subjects by using ^{18}F-FDG PET/CT (**Fig. 3**).

Prognostic Value of ^{18}F-Fluorodeoxyglucose PET–Computed Tomography in Pancreatic Adenocarcinoma

Although multiple prognostic factors have been reported in PDAC, such as serum carbohydrate antigen 19–9 (CA 19–9), as well as multiple pathologic factors, including local (T) stage,

lymphovascular invasion, lymph node (LN) metastasis, perineural invasion, and involvement of resection margin,[47,48] most of the current established predictors of outcome are inconsistent and based on findings that can only be assessed after surgical resection. For this reason, noninvasive preoperative markers are needed for risk stratification in PDAC. By finding prognostic information on pretreatment studies, therapeutic approaches can be better tailored and personalized.

Many investigators have shown correlation of ^{18}F-FDG PET/CT parameters in pretreatment studies with prognosis, in different treatment settings (**Table 2**). Sperti and colleagues[49] evaluated 60 subjects who had a preoperative FDG PET/CT, and showed that standard uptake value (SUV) was an independent predictor of survival ($P = .0002$). Schellenberg and colleagues[50] reviewed pretreatment FDG PET/CT studies of 55 subjects with locally advanced pancreatic adenocarcinoma for maximum SUV (SUVmax) and metabolic tumor burden (MTB) who were

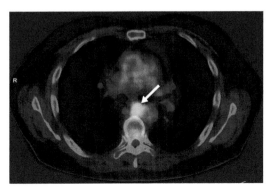

Fig. 3. ^{18}F-FDG PET/CT image of a 61-year-old man with pancreatic adenocarcinoma (not shown) and FDG avid periesophageal lymphadenopathy (*arrow*), consistent with distant metastatic disease.

Table 2
Studies evaluating the role of ^{18}F-fluorodeoxyglucose PET–computed tomography for outcome prediction in subjects with pancreatic adenocarcinoma

Study	Design	Number of Subjects	Type of Tumor	Type of Treatment	Outcome	Parameters Analyzed	Results
Sperti et al,[49] 2003	Retrospective	60	Not specified	Not specified	OS	SUV	SUV predictor for OS ($P = .0002$)
Schellenberg et al,[50] 2010	Retrospective	55	Locally advanced pancreatic adenocarcinoma	Stereotactic body radiotherapy plus gemcitabine-based chemotherapy	OS, PFS	SUVmax, MTV	SUVmax predictor for OS ($P = .03$) and PFS ($P = .03$)
Okamoto et al,[51] 2011	Retrospective	56	Resectable pancreatic adenocarcinoma	Resection ± chemoradiation	Recurrence within 6 mo after resection	SUVmax	SUVmax predictor for recurrence in 6 mo ($P = .0062$)
Choi et al,[55] 2014	Retrospective	60	Locally advanced pancreatic adenocarcinoma	Chemoradiation	OS, PFS, and LRPFS	SUVmax, MTV, and TLG	MTV, TLG and SUVmax predictive of PFS, OS and LRPFS ($P<.01$) and SUVmax predictive of PFS and LRPFS ($P<.03$)
Xu et al,[52] 2014	Retrospective	122	Resectable pancreatic adenocarcinoma	Resection ± chemoradiation	OS, PFS	SUVmax, MTV and TLG	MTV and TLG predictive of PFS and OS ($P<.008$), no correlation for SUVmax was seen
Chirindel et al,[56] 2015	Retrospective	106	All types	Surgery/chemotherapy/radiation	OS, PFS	MTV and TLG by gradient-based segmentation and fixed-threshold (50% SUVmax and SUV peak) models	SUVmax, SUVpeak and TLG associated with PFS and TLG associated with OS ($P<.04$)
Kang et al,[54] 2016	Retrospective	57	Resectable pancreatic adenocarcinoma	Resection ± chemoradiation	Recurrence	SUVmax, MTV2.5 and TLG	MTV2.5 independent predictor of tumor recurrence following margin-negative resection ($P = .034$)
Lee et al,[53] 2014	Retrospective	87	Resectable pancreatic adenocarcinoma	Resection ± chemoradiation	OS, PFS and tumor resurgence	SUVmax, MTV and TLG	MTV and TLG predictive of PFS and OS ($P<.003$) and recurrence ($P<.05$)

Abbreviations: MTV, metabolic tumor volume; SUV, standard uptake value; TLG, total lesion glycolysis.

then treated with a stereotactic body radiotherapy and a gemcitabine-based chemotherapy. They found that SUVmax was an independent predictor of OS and PFS ($P = .03$ for both). There was also a difference in median survival for high and low SUVmax (9.8 vs 15.3 months, respectively; $P<.01$) and for high and low MTB (10.1 vs 18.0 months, respectively; $P<.01$). Additionally, when clinical SUVmax cutoffs of greater than 10, 5 to 10, and less than 5 were used, median survival was 6.4, 9.5, and 17.7 months, respectively ($P<.01$). Okamoto and colleagues[51] also evaluated preoperative FDG PET/CT studies of 56 subjects with pancreatic cancer who underwent surgical resection and found that SUVmax was predictive of recurrence at 6 months ($P = .0062$).

Many studies[52–56] showed correlation of pretreatment volume-based metabolic parameters as a tumor's metabolic tumor volume (MTV) and total lesion glycolysis (TLG) for prediction of PFS and OS, as well as tumor recurrence in subjects undergoing surgical resection or chemoradiation.[52,54] Sheikhbahaei and colleagues[57] studied the prognostic value of PET/CT on therapy response assessment in subjects with locally advanced pancreatic adenocarcinoma. Forty-two subjects were included and ^{18}F-FDG PET/CT was performed in an average of 4.6 weeks after completion of chemotherapy or chemoradiation therapy. Therapy assessment ^{18}F-FDG PET/CT led to a change in the overall management of 22 (52.4%) subjects, prompting either surgical resection, adding radiation therapy, or palliative chemotherapy. SUV peak, TLG, and MTV of the post-treatment PET/CT were significant predictors of OS.

Role of PET–Computed Tomography Assessing Residual Disease and Recurrence in Pancreatic Adenocarcinoma

For patients with resectable PDAC, surgery is the treatment of choice because it is the only curative option. Most of the patients, however, have either locally advanced or metastatic disease at the time of diagnosis and are treated with chemotherapy or chemoradiation. Evaluation for residual tumor and or tumor recurrence in these patients is limited by conventional anatomic imaging such as CT and MR imaging, because postsurgical and fibrotic changes (mainly related to radiation therapy) are usually difficult to differentiate from tumor (**Fig. 4**). Moreover, tissue sampling of the areas suspicious for recurrence is difficult to obtain because pancreatic adenocarcinomas are associated with marked desmoplastic reaction.

The value of ^{18}F-FDG PET/CT for detection of suspected recurrence of PDAC after surgery compared with CT/MR imaging was evaluated in 31 subjects by Ruf and colleagues.[58] ^{18}F-FDG PET/CT detected 96% (22 of 23) and CT/MR imaging 39% (9 of 23) local recurrences and 42% (5 of 12) and 92% (11 of 12) of liver metastasis, respectively. A limitation was that the impact of these findings was not correlated with subject outcome. Sperti and colleagues[59] retrospectively evaluated 72 subjects who underwent curative resection for PDAC and who were reassessed by CT and ^{18}F-FDG PET or ^{18}F-FDG PET/CT after surgery. Conventional CT detected tumor recurrence in 35 subjects and FDG-PET in 61 subjects, and ^{18}F-FDG PET/CT changed management in 32 of 72 subjects (44.4%). However, there was no significant difference in OS between subjects with a

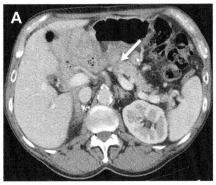
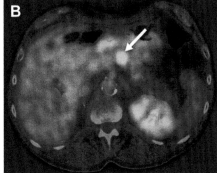

Fig. 4. A 71-year-old man with adenocarcinoma of the pancreatic head status after pancreaticoduodenectomy and adjuvant chemotherapy. Increasing serum tumor marker (Ca19-9) prompted the acquisition of contrast-enhanced CT of the abdomen (*A*), which showed indeterminate small hypodensity within the resection bed (*arrow*). ^{18}F-FDG PET/CT (*B*) showed marked increased FDG uptake at the resection bed (*arrow*), corresponding to the area of indeterminate hypodensity on prior CT, which was biopsied and proven to be tumor recurrence at the resection bed.

positive CT and those who were indeterminate on CT and positive on ^{18}F-FDG PET/CT.

For subjects undergoing chemoradiation, residual disease was detected by ^{18}F-FDG PET/CT in 5 of 15 subjects, compared with none detected by CT in a study of Bang and colleagues.[60] Yoshioka and colleagues[61] also suggested that ^{18}F-FDG PET/CT can detect response to treatment before CT; however, investigators had a small sample of only 10 subjects. More studies are needed to assess the usefulness of FDG PET/CT in subjects with pancreatic adenocarcinoma undergoing chemoradiation.

Given that FDG is a nonspecific marker of glucose metabolism, other factors, such as postsurgical inflammatory changes, response to radiation therapy, and stent placement, can increase the number of false-positive studies and, for this reason, it is recommended to perform FDG PET/CT 6 weeks after surgery.[58,61]

In summary, although FDG PET/CT was is potentially effective to detect residual or recurrent disease, more studies are needed to prove its impact on patient survival.

Novel PET–Computed Tomography Tracer in Pancreatic Adenocarcinoma

There is an increasing interest in new tracers for imaging pancreatic adenocarcinoma, focusing on improving the diagnosis, prognostic value, and evaluation of response to treatment. Imaging biomarkers can provide not only spatial information and heterogeneity of the entirety of the tumor but also noninvasive longitudinal analysis. However, these tracers have yet to accurately reflect the underlying biological process.

Imaging of cell proliferation: ^{18}F-fluorothymidine PET–computed tomography

The rate of proliferation in cancer cells has been proved to correlate with prognosis and outcome in many cancers.[62,63] ^{18}F-fluorothymidine (FLT), a thymidine analogue that is monophosphorylated by thymidine kinase 1 (TK1), leading to intracellular trapping, has been proposed as an imaging biomarker of tumor proliferation. TK1 activity is increased during phase S of cell cycle, translating into a proliferation marker. Also, Ki-67, the gold-standard immunohistochemical marker for tumor proliferation, has shown a strong spatial correlation with FLT uptake for brain, lung, and breast cancer.[64]

The added value of ^{18}F-FLT PET/CT compared with ^{18}F-FDG PET/CT is the elimination of uptake confounders related to hypoxia or inflammation, which can be seen on ^{18}F-FDG PET/CT. This is especially important on the assessment of

response to treatment, increasing specificity and as a valuable tool in the development of anticancer therapies.

Herrmann and colleagues[65] investigated the ability of ^{18}F-FLT PET to differentiate malignant (PDAC) from benign pancreatic lesions in 31 subjects with indeterminate lesions. They found that the 10 benign lesions were negative on FLT PET (specificity of 100%) and 15 of the 21 malignant tumors were positive (sensitivity of 71.4%), and the tumors missed were either well-differentiated or small tumors. The uptake was significantly higher in malignant compared with benign tumors ($P = .001$).

On a subsequent larger study, Herrmann and colleagues[66] also compared the diagnostic accuracy of ^{18}F-FLT PET to ^{18}F-FDG PET or PET/CT in 42 subjects with a pancreatic suspicious mass or chronic pancreatitis. FLT had a 70% sensitivity and 75% specificity, compared with 92% and 50% for FDG, respectively. Of note, FLT were PET-only studies, which may have limited the evaluation by lack of anatomic references.

Recently, Challapalli and colleagues[67] evaluated 20 subjects with advanced pancreatic carcinoma with dynamic ^{18}F-FLT PT/CT before and 3 weeks after the first cycle of gemcitabine-based chemotherapy. Primary tumors and metastasis were analyzed using kinetic spatial filtering to increase lesion detectability. SUVmax at 60 minutes after tracer injection was significantly higher in subjects with disease progression ($P = .04$).

Early detection of response to treatment is probably going to be the main role of ^{18}F-FLT-PET/CT in pancreatic cancer, as it has shown for other tumors. Because the degree of uptake is relatively low on lesions and physiologic bowel uptake can be seen, an anatomic image is necessary for correct interpretation. More studies are needed to investigate the correlation of FLT uptake in PDAC with histologic proliferation markers.[68]

Textural Analysis

There is a growing interest for quantification of intratumoral heterogeneity, which, at a molecular level, can be related to treatment failure and drug resistance.[69] Hyun and colleagues[70] reported the role of intratumoral heterogeneity texture analysis by ^{18}F-FDG PET to predict outcome in subjects with PDAC. A total of 137 primary lesions were analyzed in pretreatment ^{18}F-FDG PET with first-order and higher-order textural features, and conventional PET parameters were also measured. Higher entropy (hazard ratio [HR] 5.59, $P = .028$) was independently associated with worse survival.

Mena and colleagues[71] also analyzed the factors that contribute to standardize uptake time and segmentation methods for MTV and intratumoral heterogeneity index by using dual-time point (1 hour, early, and 2 hours, delayed) images in pretreatment ^{18}F-FDG PET/CT in 71 subjects with pancreatic adenocarcinomas. As well as the dual-time point, a comparison of automated PET segmentation method and 50% SUVmax threshold segmentation methods was performed. They found that MTV values remained consistent between early and delayed imaging when using the gradient PET segmentation method ($P = .086$), whereas statistically significant change was seen when using 50% SUVmax threshold segmentation ($P<.001$). Tumor heterogeneity showed statistically significant differences between early and delayed time points ($P<.001$) when using the gradient segmentation and remained stable between early and delayed when using the 50% SUVmax threshold segmentation ($P = .148$).

A novel metric for tumor quantification was developed by Rahmim and colleagues,[72] named generalized effective total uptake (gETU), which encompasses different FDG PET metrics, such as SUVmax, TLG, and MTV, with different emphases on PET uptake versus volume. The gETU was evaluated for OS predictor in 72 subjects with locally advanced pancreatic adenocarcinoma. An improved HR value was found for gETU compared with other individual parameters, with a significant independent value for OS prediction ($P = .0067$).

PANCREATIC NEUROENDOCRINE TUMORS
Diagnostic Studies

Pancreatic NETs are rare tumors (1% of all pancreatic cancers) that arise in the endocrine tissues of the pancreas (islet cell tumors). These tumors have a broad spectrum of aggressiveness, which is related to different factors, including the grade of malignancy, tumor burden, and presence of metastases, among others.[73] Most pancreatic NETs are nonfunctioning and not associated with a hormonal syndrome, but a minority can secrete a broad variety of peptide hormones.

SSTRs are overexpressed in the cell surface of pancreatic NETs,[74,75] the most abundant subtype being SSTR2.[76] For this reason, gamma camera imaging with a radiolabeled form of the somatostatin analogue [111]in-DTPA-octreotide can be used for diagnosis of NETs by binding SSTR2 and SSTR4.[77,78] The sensitivity of SSTR scintigraphy is reported in the range of 82% to 95%, which is superior when compared with pure anatomic imaging methods, such as CT, MR imaging, and endoscopic US, for identification of islet cell tumors, carcinoids, and their metastases.[79–85] Of note, the diagnosis of insulinomas is limited, given the low SSTR expression in these tumors.[86] The addition of SPECT associated with CT provides hybrid anatomic (CT) and functional (SPECT) imaging, enhancing the specificity and increasing the diagnostic confidence for tumor localization[87,88] (**Fig. 5**).

PET using ^{68}Ga-labeled somatostatin analogues has been more recently used for diagnosis of NETs, enabling better sensitivity and spatial resolution.[74,89–92] Currently, there are no clinical reports to support preferential use of one specific analogue (ie, DOTATOC [DOTA-Tyl[3]-octreotide], DOTANOC [DOTA-Nal[3]-octreotide], DOTATATE [DOTA-Tyr[3]-octreotate]) over the other.[93] ^{68}Ga-DOTATATE PET/CT was shown to be highly accurate for detection in subjects with suspected NETs due to clinical symptoms, elevated levels of tumor markers, or

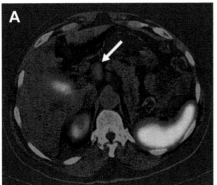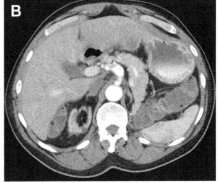

Fig. 5. A 65-year-old woman with history of diarrhea and anxiety had an SPECT/CT octreoscan performed that showed a focal area of uptake (*arrow*) in the region of the pancreatic head (*A*). She had a concurrent CT of the abdomen that was not able to localize the lesion (*B*). The lesion was biopsied by endoscopic US-guided procedure, confirming a NET.

indeterminate findings for NET in alternative imaging, supporting its use in clinical routine diagnostics.[94]

Buchmann and colleagues.[74] showed the benefit of using 68Ga-DOTATOC PET/CT compared with 111In-pentetreotide SPECT/CT, with the most obvious superiority represented by detection of additional lungs and skeleton metastases by 68Ga-DOTATOC PET. Other investigators also described the benefit of 68Ga-DOTA-labeled somatostatin analogues in the detection of unsuspected bone lesions, although one study reported a significantly low incidence of bone lesions in subjects with pancreatic NETs.[95]

Frilling and colleagues[96] reported significant impact of 68Ga-DOTATOC PET/CT findings compared with CT and/or MR imaging alone in 31 (59.6%) of the 52 subjects studied with pancreatic NETs. Ilhan and colleagues[97] stated that the additional information provided by preoperative 68Ga-DOTATATE PET/CT significantly changed surgical management in one-third of subjects with NETs of the pancreas.

A pilot study from Beiderwellen and colleagues[98] demonstrated the potential of 68Ga-DOTATOC PET/MR imaging in subjects with gastroenteropancreatic NETs, with advantages in the characterization of abdominal lesions. However, there were some limitations related to identification of lung metastases and sclerotic bone lesions.

The role of 18F-FDG PET/CT for detection of pancreatic NETs has been described by Cingarlini and colleagues,[99] who compared it with 68Ga-DOTATOC PET/CT. A total of 35 subjects with biopsied proven neuroendocrine pancreatic cancer were classified in grade 1 and grade 2 tumors based on the World Health Organization classification, with 28.6% grade 1 and 71.4% grade 2 tumors. 68Ga-DOTATOC PET/CT showed

expected high sensitivity (94.3%) in detecting grade 1 and 2 pancreatic NETs, and FDG PET/CT had a high positive predictive value (90.5%) for grade 2 tumors, with a potential role in prognosis and risk stratification (**Fig. 6**).

The prognostic value of 18F-FDG PET/CT for patients with pancreatic NETs was investigated by Kim and colleagues[100] in 20 subjects with pretreatment 18F-FDG PET/CT using volumetric parameters. MTV (HR 10.859, $P = .031$) was found to be a significant independent predictor of OS. Additionally, Ambrosini and colleagues[101] showed that 68Ga-DOTANOC high SUVmax was a risk factor for tumor progression (HR 3.09; $P = .003$) in 43 subjects.

Peptide Receptor Radioligand Therapy

Radiolabeled somatostatin analogues can be used for therapy in patients with disease refractory to medical therapy with tumors that express SSTRs.[102–107] Yttrium-90 (90Y) and Lutetium-177 (177Lu) are the most frequently used radionuclides, with different emitted particles, energies, and tissue penetration.[107]

The largest study with 90Y-DOTATOC[106] studied 1109 subjects with metastatic gastroenteropancreatic NET who presented tumor uptake on pretreatment SSTR scintigraphy. Subjects were treated with an initial dose, which was repeated if there was not tumor progression or toxicity (median of 2 doses, ranging from 1 to 10).

A total of 378 (34.1%) subjects showed morphologic response; 172 (15.5%), biochemical response; and 329 (29.7%), clinical response. The median survival from diagnosis was 94.6 months, with longer survival correlating with responses by any of this criteria.

For 177Lu-DOTATATE treatment, 310 subjects with gastroenteropancreatic NET were evaluated

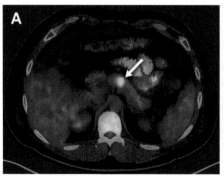
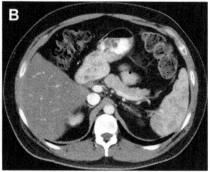

Fig. 6. A 33-year-old man with an enlarging mass in the right axillary region (not shown) had a biopsy that showed a NET. Staging 18F-FDG PET/CT also detected a lesion (*arrow*) in the pancreas (*A*), also biopsy-proven NET, which was not visualized on the staging CT (*B*).

in a study from Kwekkeboom and colleagues[103] Subjects were treated with a median of 4 treatment cycles. An objective response rate of 30% was reported, with higher response rates in pancreatic NET, ranging from 36% for nonfunctioning tumors, to approximately 40 to 60% for functioning gastrinomas, insulinomas, and VIPomas.

A nonrandomized study suggested that 177Lu-DOTATATE outperforms 90Y DOTATATE.[107] A total of 450 subjects with pancreatic or gastrointestinal NET were treated with 177Lu-DOTATATE (54%), 90Y DOTATATE (17%), or combined therapy (29%). The progression-free period was 27 months for 90Y DOTATATE alone, 40 months for 177Lu-DOTATATE, and 50 months for combined therapy.

Recently, the NETTER-1 trial (Neuroendocrine Tumors Therapy), a randomized phase 3 trial for subjects with advanced midgut NET who have had disease progression during first-line somatostatin analogue therapy assigned 229 subjects with well-differentiated metastatic midgut NETs to receive either ^{177}Lu-DOTATATE or high-dose octreotide.

A total of 116 subjects received ^{177}Lu-Dotatate at a dose of 7.4 GBq every 8 weeks (4 intravenous infusions plus octreotide long-acting repeatable [LAR]) and 113 subjects received octreotide LAR alone administered intramuscularly at a dose of 60 mg every 4 weeks. The primary analysis showed that the estimated rate of PFS at 20 months was 65.2% (95% CI 50.0–76.8) in the ^{177}Lu-Dotatate group and 10.8% (95% CI 3.5–23.0) in the octreotide LAR group. The interim analysis for OS showed 14 deaths in ^{177}Lu-Dotatate group and 26 in octreotide LAR group ($P<.004$). There was a small rate of side-effects with neutropenia (1%), thrombocytopenia (2%), and lymphopenia (9%) in the ^{177}Lu-Dotatate group compared with none in the octreotide group. The study concluded that treatment with ^{177}Lu-Dotatate is superior to octreotide LAR treatment in subjects with advanced midgut NETs by showing a longer PFS, higher response rate, and preliminary evidence of OS benefit, with less than 10% of clinically significant myelosupression.[108]

SUMMARY

Imaging studies have a very important role in detection, staging, evaluation of response to treatment and prognosis prediction in patients with pancreatic adenocarcinoma and NETs. Because many molecular pathways are involved in the development and maintenance of adenocarcinoma cells in the pancreas, a specific agent to target a given mechanism has not been developed yet. The overexpression of SSTR on the surface of the cancerous cells of NETs facilitated the development of imaging and therapy modalities that are highly specific, enabling theranostics and providing survival benefits to patients with NETs.

REFERENCES

1. Siegel RL, Miller KD, Jemal A. Cancer statistics, 2017. CA Cancer J Clin 2017;67(1):7–30.
2. Von Hoff DD, Ramanathan RK, Borad MJ, et al. Gemcitabine plus nab-paclitaxel is an active regimen in patients with advanced pancreatic cancer: a phase I/II trial. J Clin Oncol 2011; 29(34):4548–54.
3. Von Hoff DD, Ervin T, Arena FP, et al. Increased survival in pancreatic cancer with nab-paclitaxel plus gemcitabine. N Engl J Med 2013;369(18): 1691–703.
4. Goldstein D, El-Maraghi RH, Hammel P, et al. nab-Paclitaxel plus gemcitabine for metastatic pancreatic cancer: long-term survival from a phase III trial. J Natl Cancer Inst 2015;107(2) [pii:dju413].
5. Ychou M, Desseigne F, Guimbaud R, et al. Randomized phase II trial comparing folfirinox (5FU/leucovorin [LV], irinotecan [I]and oxaliplatin [O]) vs gemcitabine (G) as first-line treatment for metastatic pancreatic adenocarcinoma (MPA). First results of the ACCORD 11 trial. J Clin Oncol 2007; 25:210 [abstract: 4516].
6. Waddell N, Pajic M, Patch AM, et al. Whole genomes redefine the mutational landscape of pancreatic cancer. Nature 2015;518(7540):495–501.
7. Jones S, Zhang X, Parsons DW, et al. Core signaling pathways in human pancreatic cancers revealed by global genomic analyses. Science 2008;321(5897):1801–6.
8. Nandy D, Mukhopadhyay D. Growth factor mediated signaling in pancreatic pathogenesis. Cancers (Basel) 2011;3(1):841–71.
9. Samuel N, Hudson TJ. The molecular and cellular heterogeneity of pancreatic ductal adenocarcinoma. Nat Rev Gastroenterol Hepatol 2011;9(2): 77–87.
10. Troiani T, Martinelli E, Capasso A, et al. Targeting EGFR in pancreatic cancer treatment. Curr Drug Targets 2012;13(6):802–10.
11. Ciardiello F, Tortora G. EGFR antagonists in cancer treatment. N Engl J Med 2008;358(11):1160–74.
12. Modjtahedi H, Dean C. The receptor for EGF and its ligands - expression, prognostic value and target for therapy in cancer (review). Int J Oncol 1994;4(2):277–96.
13. Salomon DS, Brandt R, Ciardiello F, et al. Epidermal growth factor-related peptides and their

receptors in human malignancies. Crit Rev Oncol Hematol 1995;19(3):183–232.

14. Cohenuram M, Saif MW. Epidermal growth factor receptor inhibition strategies in pancreatic cancer: past, present and the future. JOP 2007;8(1):4–15.

15. Philip PA, Benedetti J, Corless CL, et al. Phase III study comparing gemcitabine plus cetuximab versus gemcitabine in patients with advanced pancreatic adenocarcinoma: Southwest Oncology Group-directed intergroup trial S0205. J Clin Oncol 2010;28(22):3605–10.

16. Moore MJ, Goldstein D, Hamm J, et al. Erlotinib plus gemcitabine compared with gemcitabine alone in patients with advanced pancreatic cancer: a phase III trial of the National Cancer Institute of Canada Clinical Trials Group. J Clin Oncol 2007; 25(15):1960–6.

17. Jeltsch M, Kaipainen A, Joukov V, et al. Hyperplasia of lymphatic vessels in VEGF-C transgenic mice. Science 1997;276(5317):1423–5.

18. Ferrara N. Role of vascular endothelial growth factor in the regulation of angiogenesis. Kidney Int 1999;56(3):794–814.

19. Shibuya M, Yamaguchi S, Yamane A, et al. Nucleotide sequence and expression of a novel human receptor-type tyrosine kinase gene (flt) closely related to the fms family. Oncogene 1990;5(4): 519–24.

20. Fischer C, Mazzone M, Jonckx B, et al. FLT1 and its ligands VEGFB and PlGF: drug targets for anti-angiogenic therapy? Nat Rev Cancer 2008;8(12): 942–56.

21. Kindler HL, Friberg G, Singh DA, et al. Phase II trial of bevacizumab plus gemcitabine in patients with advanced pancreatic cancer. J Clin Oncol 2005; 23(31):8033–40.

22. Kindler HL, Niedzwiecki D, Hollis D, et al. Gemcitabine plus bevacizumab compared with gemcitabine plus placebo in patients with advanced pancreatic cancer: phase III trial of the Cancer and Leukemia Group B (CALGB 80303). J Clin Oncol 2010;28(22):3617–22.

23. Van Cutsem E, Vervenne WL, Bennouna J, et al. Phase III trial of bevacizumab in combination with gemcitabine and erlotinib in patients with metastatic pancreatic cancer. J Clin Oncol 2009;27(13): 2231–7.

24. Kanda M, Matthaei H, Wu J, et al. Presence of somatic mutations in most early-stage pancreatic intraepithelial neoplasia. Gastroenterology 2012; 142(4):730–3.e9.

25. Collins MA, Bednar F, Zhang Y, et al. Oncogenic Kras is required for both the initiation and maintenance of pancreatic cancer in mice. J Clin Invest 2012;122(2):639–53.

26. Bournet B, Buscail C, Muscari F, et al. Targeting KRAS for diagnosis, prognosis, and treatment of pancreatic cancer: hopes and realities. Eur J Cancer 2016;54:75–83.

27. Kauhanen SP, Komar G, Seppanen MP, et al. A prospective diagnostic accuracy study of 18F-fluorodeoxyglucose positron emission tomography/computed tomography, multidetector row computed tomography, and magnetic resonance imaging in primary diagnosis and staging of pancreatic cancer. Ann Surg 2009;250(6):957–63.

28. Heinrich S, Goerres GW, Schafer M, et al. Positron emission tomography/computed tomography influences on the management of resectable pancreatic cancer and its cost-effectiveness. Ann Surg 2005;242(2):235–43.

29. Schick V, Franzius C, Beyna T, et al. Diagnostic impact of 18F-FDG PET-CT evaluating solid pancreatic lesions versus endosonography, endoscopic retrograde cholangio-pancreatography with intraductal ultrasonography and abdominal ultrasound. Eur J Nucl Med Mol Imaging 2008; 35(10):1775–85.

30. Buchs NC, Buhler L, Bucher P, et al. Value of contrast-enhanced 18F-fluorodeoxyglucose positron emission tomography/computed tomography in detection and presurgical assessment of pancreatic cancer: a prospective study. J Gastroenterol Hepatol 2011;26(4):657–62.

31. Lemke AJ, Niehues SM, Hosten N, et al. Retrospective digital image fusion of multidetector CT and 18F-FDG PET: clinical value in pancreatic lesions–a prospective study with 104 patients. J Nucl Med 2004;45(8):1279–86.

32. Koyama K, Okamura T, Kawabe J, et al. Diagnostic usefulness of FDG PET for pancreatic mass lesions. Ann Nucl Med 2001;15(3):217–24.

33. Santhosh S, Mittal BR, Bhasin D, et al. Role of (18) F-fluorodeoxyglucose positron emission tomography/computed tomography in the characterization of pancreatic masses: experience from tropics. J Gastroenterol Hepatol 2013;28(2):255–61.

34. Rose DM, Delbeke D, Beauchamp RD, et al. 18Fluorodeoxyglucose-positron emission tomography in the management of patients with suspected pancreatic cancer. Ann Surg 1999;229(5):729–37 [discussion: 737–8].

35. Diederichs CG, Staib L, Vogel J, et al. Values and limitations of 18F-fluorodeoxyglucose-positron-emission tomography with preoperative evaluation of patients with pancreatic masses. Pancreas 2000;20(2):109–16.

36. Matsumoto I, Shirakawa S, Shinzeki M, et al. 18-Fluorodeoxyglucose positron emission tomography does not aid in diagnosis of pancreatic ductal adenocarcinoma. Clin Gastroenterol Hepatol 2013;11(6):712–8.

37. Strobel O, Buchler MW. Pancreatic cancer: FDG-PET is not useful in early pancreatic cancer

diagnosis. Nat Rev Gastroenterol Hepatol 2013; 10(4):203–5.

38. Shreve PD. Focal fluorine-18 fluorodeoxyglucose accumulation in inflammatory pancreatic disease. Eur J Nucl Med 1998;25(3):259–64.

39. Zimny M, Buell U, Diederichs CG, et al. False-positive FDG PET in patients with pancreatic masses: an issue of proper patient selection? Eur J Nucl Med 1998;25(9):1352.

40. Higashi T, Saga T, Nakamoto Y, et al. Diagnosis of pancreatic cancer using fluorine-18 fluorodeoxyglucose positron emission tomography (FDG PET) –usefulness and limitations in "clinical reality". Ann Nucl Med 2003;17(4):261–79.

41. Wakabayashi H, Nishiyama Y, Otani T, et al. Role of 18F-fluorodeoxyglucose positron emission tomography imaging in surgery for pancreatic cancer. World J Gastroenterol 2008;14(1):64–9.

42. Soriano A, Castells A, Ayuso C, et al. Preoperative staging and tumor resectability assessment of pancreatic cancer: prospective study comparing endoscopic ultrasonography, helical computed tomography, magnetic resonance imaging, and angiography. Am J Gastroenterol 2004;99(3): 492–501.

43. Wang XY, Yang F, Jin C, et al. The value of 18F-FDG positron emission tomography/computed tomography on the pre-operative staging and the management of patients with pancreatic carcinoma. Hepatogastroenterology 2014;61(135):2102–9.

44. Kim MJ, Lee KH, Lee KT, et al. The value of positron emission tomography/computed tomography for evaluating metastatic disease in patients with pancreatic cancer. Pancreas 2012;41(6): 897–903.

45. Asagi A, Ohta K, Nasu J, et al. Utility of contrast-enhanced FDG-PET/CT in the clinical management of pancreatic cancer: impact on diagnosis, staging, evaluation of treatment response, and detection of recurrence. Pancreas 2013;42(1):11–9.

46. Chang JS, Choi SH, Lee Y, et al. Clinical usefulness of ^{18}F-fluorodeoxyglucose-positron emission tomography in patients with locally advanced pancreatic cancer planned to undergo concurrent chemoradiation therapy. Int J Radiat Oncol Biol Phys 2014;90(1):126–33.

47. Lewis R, Drebin JA, Callery MP, et al. A contemporary analysis of survival for resected pancreatic ductal adenocarcinoma. HPB (Oxford) 2013;15(1):49–60.

48. Kato K, Yamada S, Sugimoto H, et al. Prognostic factors for survival after extended pancreatectomy for pancreatic head cancer: influence of resection margin status on survival. Pancreas 2009;38(6): 605–12.

49. Sperti C, Pasquali C, Chierichetti F, et al. 18-Fluorodeoxyglucose positron emission tomography in predicting survival of patients with pancreatic carcinoma. J Gastrointest Surg 2003;7(8):953–9 [discussion: 959–60].

50. Schellenberg D, Quon A, Minn AY, et al. 18Fluorodeoxyglucose PET is prognostic of progression-free and overall survival in locally advanced pancreas cancer treated with stereotactic radiotherapy. Int J Radiat Oncol Biol Phys 2010;77(5): 1420–5.

51. Okamoto K, Koyama I, Miyazawa M, et al. Preoperative 18[F]-fluorodeoxyglucose positron emission tomography/computed tomography predicts early recurrence after pancreatic cancer resection. Int J Clin Oncol 2011;16(1):39–44.

52. Xu HX, Chen T, Wang WQ, et al. Metabolic tumour burden assessed by (1)(8)F-FDG PET/CT associated with serum CA19-9 predicts pancreatic cancer outcome after resection. Eur J Nucl Med Mol Imaging 2014;41(6):1093–102.

53. Lee JW, Kang CM, Choi HJ, et al. Prognostic value of metabolic tumor volume and total lesion glycolysis on preoperative (1)(8)F-FDG PET/CT in patients with pancreatic cancer. J Nucl Med 2014;55(6):898–904.

54. Kang CM, Lee SH, Hwang HK, et al. Preoperative volume-based PET parameter, MTV2.5, as a potential Surrogate marker for tumor biology and recurrence in resected pancreatic cancer. Medicine 2016;95(9):e2595.

55. Choi HJ, Lee JW, Kang B, et al. Prognostic significance of volume-based FDG PET/CT parameters in patients with locally advanced pancreatic cancer treated with chemoradiation therapy. Yonsei Med J 2014;55(6):1498–506.

56. Chirindel A, Alluri KC, Chaudhry MA, et al. Prognostic value of FDG PET/CT-derived parameters in pancreatic adenocarcinoma at initial PET/CT staging. AJR Am J Roentgenol 2015;204(5):1093–9.

57. Sheikhbahaei S, Wray R, Young B, et al. 18F-FDG-PET/CT therapy assessment of locally advanced pancreatic adenocarcinoma: impact on management and utilization of quantitative parameters for patient survival prediction. Nucl Med Commun 2016;37(3):231–8.

58. Ruf J, Lopez Hanninen E, Oettle H, et al. Detection of recurrent pancreatic cancer: comparison of FDG-PET with CT/MRI. Pancreatology 2005; 5(2–3):266–72.

59. Sperti C, Pasquali C, Bissoli S, et al. Tumor relapse after pancreatic cancer resection is detected earlier by 18-FDG PET than by CT. J Gastrointest Surg 2010;14(1):131–40.

60. Bang S, Chung HW, Park SW, et al. The clinical usefulness of 18-fluorodeoxyglucose positron emission tomography in the differential diagnosis, staging, and response evaluation after concurrent chemoradiotherapy for pancreatic cancer. J Clin Gastroenterol 2006;40(10):923–9.

61. Yoshioka M, Sato T, Furuya T, et al. Role of positron emission tomography with 2-deoxy-2-[18F]fluoro-D-glucose in evaluating the effects of arterial infusion chemotherapy and radiotherapy on pancreatic cancer. J Gastroenterol 2004;39(1):50–5.

62. Martin B, Paesmans M, Mascaux C, et al. Ki-67 expression and patients survival in lung cancer: systematic review of the literature with meta-analysis. Br J Cancer 2004;91(12):2018–25.

63. de Azambuja E, Cardoso F, de Castro G Jr, et al. Ki-67 as prognostic marker in early breast cancer: a meta-analysis of published studies involving 12,155 patients. Br J Cancer 2007;96(10):1504–13.

64. Chalkidou A, Landau DB, Odell EW, et al. Correlation between Ki-67 immunohistochemistry and 18F-fluorothymidine uptake in patients with cancer: a systematic review and meta-analysis. Eur J Cancer 2012;48(18):3499–513.

65. Herrmann K, Eckel F, Schmidt S, et al. In vivo characterization of proliferation for discriminating cancer from pancreatic pseudotumors. J Nucl Med 2008;49(9):1437–44.

66. Herrmann K, Erkan M, Dobritz M, et al. Comparison of 3'-deoxy-3'-[(1)(8)F]fluorothymidine positron emission tomography (FLT PET) and FDG PET/CT for the detection and characterization of pancreatic tumours. Eur J Nucl Med Mol Imaging 2012;39(5):846–51.

67. Challapalli A, Barwick T, Pearson RA, et al. 3'-Deoxy-3'-^{18}F-fluorothymidine positron emission tomography as an early predictor of disease progression in patients with advanced and metastatic pancreatic cancer. Eur J Nucl Med Mol Imaging 2015;42(6):831–40.

68. Lamarca A, Asselin MC, Manoharan P, et al. 18F-FLT PET imaging of cellular proliferation in pancreatic cancer. Crit Rev Oncol Hematol 2016;99:158–69.

69. Gerlinger M, Rowan AJ, Horswell S, et al. Intratumor heterogeneity and branched evolution revealed by multiregion sequencing. N Engl J Med 2012;366(10):883–92.

70. Hyun SH, Kim HS, Choi SH, et al. Intratumoral heterogeneity of (18)F-FDG uptake predicts survival in patients with pancreatic ductal adenocarcinoma. Eur J Nucl Med Mol Imaging 2016;43(8):1461–8.

71. Mena E, Sheikhbahaei S, Taghipour M, et al. 18F-FDG PET/CT metabolic tumor volume and intratumoral heterogeneity in pancreatic adenocarcinomas: impact of dual-time point and segmentation methods. Clin Nucl Med 2017;42(1):e16–21.

72. Rahmim A, Schmidtlein CR, Jackson A, et al. A novel metric for quantification of homogeneous and heterogeneous tumors in PET for enhanced clinical outcome prediction. Phys Med Biol 2016;61(1):227–42.

73. Yao JC, Hassan M, Phan A, et al. One hundred years after "carcinoid": epidemiology of and prognostic factors for neuroendocrine tumors in 35,825 cases in the United States. J Clin Oncol 2008;26(18):3063–72.

74. Buchmann I, Henze M, Engelbrecht S, et al. Comparison of 68Ga-DOTATOC PET and 111In-DTPAOC (Octreoscan) SPECT in patients with neuroendocrine tumours. Eur J Nucl Med Mol Imaging 2007;34(10):1617–26.

75. Treglia G, Castaldi P, Rindi G, et al. Diagnostic performance of Gallium-68 somatostatin receptor PET and PET/CT in patients with thoracic and gastroenteropancreatic neuroendocrine tumours: a meta-analysis. Endocrine 2012;42(1):80–7.

76. Hoyer D, Bell GI, Berelowitz M, et al. Classification and nomenclature of somatostatin receptors. Trends Pharmacol Sci 1995;16(3):86–8.

77. Krenning EP, Kwekkeboom DJ, Bakker WH, et al. Somatostatin receptor scintigraphy with [111In-DTPA-D-Phe1]- and [123I-Tyr3]-octreotide: the Rotterdam experience with more than 1000 patients. Eur J Nucl Med 1993;20(8):716–31.

78. Kwekkeboom DJ, Krenning EP. Somatostatin receptor imaging. Semin Nucl Med 2002;32(2):84–91.

79. Alexander HR, Fraker DL, Norton JA, et al. Prospective study of somatostatin receptor scintigraphy and its effect on operative outcome in patients with Zollinger-Ellison syndrome. Ann Surg 1998;228(2):228–38.

80. Cadiot G, Lebtahi R, Sarda L, et al. Preoperative detection of duodenal gastrinomas and peripancreatic lymph nodes by somatostatin receptor scintigraphy. Groupe D'etude Du Syndrome De Zollinger-Ellison. Gastroenterology 1996;111(4):845–54.

81. de Kerviler E, Cadiot G, Lebtahi R, et al. Somatostatin receptor scintigraphy in forty-eight patients with the Zollinger-Ellison syndrome. GRESZE: Groupe d'Etude du Syndrome de Zollinger-Ellison. Eur J Nucl Med 1994;21(11):1191–7.

82. Gibril F, Reynolds JC, Doppman JL, et al. Somatostatin receptor scintigraphy: its sensitivity compared with that of other imaging methods in detecting primary and metastatic gastrinomas. A prospective study. Ann Intern Med 1996;125(1):26–34.

83. Jensen RT, Gibril F, Termanini B. Definition of the role of somatostatin receptor scintigraphy in gastrointestinal neuroendocrine tumor localization. Yale J Biol Med 1997;70(5–6):481–500.

84. Termanini B, Gibril F, Reynolds JC, et al. Value of somatostatin receptor scintigraphy: a prospective study in gastrinoma of its effect on clinical management. Gastroenterology 1997;112(2):335–47.

85. Joseph S, Wang YZ, Boudreaux JP, et al. Neuroendocrine tumors: current recommendations for diagnosis and surgical management. Endocrinol Metab Clin North Am 2011;40(1):205–31, x.

86. McKenna LR, Edil BH. Update on pancreatic neuroendocrine tumors. Gland Surg 2014;3(4):258–75.

87. Krausz Y, Keidar Z, Kogan I, et al. SPECT/CT hybrid imaging with 111In-pentetreotide in assessment of neuroendocrine tumours. Clin Endocrinol 2003;59(5):565–73.

88. Even-Sapir E, Keidar Z, Sachs J, et al. The new technology of combined transmission and emission tomography in evaluation of endocrine neoplasms. J Nucl Med 2001;42(7):998–1004.

89. Lee I, Paeng JC, Lee SJ, et al. Comparison of diagnostic sensitivity and quantitative indices between (68)Ga-DOTATOC PET/CT and (111)In-Pentetreotide SPECT/CT in neuroendocrine tumors: a preliminary report. Nucl Med Mol Imaging 2015;49(4):284–90.

90. Schreiter NF, Bartels AM, Froeling V, et al. Searching for primaries in patients with neuroendocrine tumors (NET) of unknown primary and clinically suspected NET: evaluation of Ga-68 DOTATOC PET/CT and In-111 DTPA octreotide SPECT/CT. Radiol Oncol 2014;48(4):339–47.

91. Schmid-Tannwald C, Schmid-Tannwald CM, Morelli JN, et al. Comparison of abdominal MRI with diffusion-weighted imaging to 68Ga-DOTATATE PET/CT in detection of neuroendocrine tumors of the pancreas. Eur J Nucl Med Mol Imaging 2013;40(6):897–907.

92. Sharma P, Arora S, Dhull VS, et al. Evaluation of (68)Ga-DOTANOC PET/CT imaging in a large exclusive population of pancreatic neuroendocrine tumors. Abdom Imaging 2015;40(2):299–309.

93. Ambrosini V, Nanni C, Fanti S. The use of gallium-68 labeled somatostatin receptors in PET/CT imaging. PET Clin 2014;9(3):323–9.

94. Haug AR, Cindea-Drimus R, Auernhammer CJ, et al. The role of 68Ga-DOTATATE PET/CT in suspected neuroendocrine tumors. J Nucl Med 2012;53(11):1686–92.

95. Kunikowska J, Pawlak D, Kolasa A, et al. A frequency and semiquantitative analysis of pathological 68Ga DOTATATE PET/CT uptake by primary site-dependent neuroendocrine tumor metastasis. Clin Nucl Med 2014;39(10):855–61.

96. Frilling A, Sotiropoulos GC, Radtke A, et al. The impact of 68Ga-DOTATOC positron emission tomography/computed tomography on the multimodal management of patients with neuroendocrine tumors. Ann Surg 2010;252(5):850–6.

97. Ilhan H, Fendler WP, Cyran CC, et al. Impact of (68)Ga-DOTATATE PET/CT on the surgical management of primary neuroendocrine tumors of the pancreas or ileum. Ann Surg Oncol 2015;22(1):164–71.

98. Beiderwellen KJ, Poeppel TD, Hartung-Knemeyer V, et al. Simultaneous 68Ga-DOTATOC PET/MRI in patients with gastroenteropancreatic neuroendocrine tumors: initial results. Invest Radiol 2013;48(5):273–9.

99. Cingarlini S, Ortolani S, Salgarello M, et al. Role of combined 68Ga-DOTATOC and 18F-FDG positron emission tomography/computed tomography in the diagnostic workup of pancreas neuroendocrine tumors: implications for managing surgical decisions. Pancreas 2017;46(1):42–7.

100. Kim HS, Choi JY, Choi DW, et al. Prognostic value of volume-based metabolic parameters measured by (18)F-FDG PET/CT of pancreatic neuroendocrine tumors. Nucl Med Mol Imaging 2014;48(3):180–6.

101. Ambrosini V, Campana D, Polverari G, et al. Prognostic value of 68Ga-DOTANOC PET/CT SUVmax in patients with neuroendocrine tumors of the pancreas. J Nucl Med 2015;56(12):1843–8.

102. Kwekkeboom DJ, Bakker WH, Kam BL, et al. Treatment of patients with gastro-entero-pancreatic (GEP) tumours with the novel radiolabelled somatostatin analogue [177Lu-DOTA(0),Tyr3]octreotate. Eur J Nucl Med Mol Imaging 2003;30(3):417–22.

103. Kwekkeboom DJ, de Herder WW, Kam BL, et al. Treatment with the radiolabeled somatostatin analog [177 Lu-DOTA 0,Tyr3]octreotate: toxicity, efficacy, and survival. J Clin Oncol 2008;26(13):2124–30.

104. Waldherr C, Pless M, Maecke HR, et al. Tumor response and clinical benefit in neuroendocrine tumors after 7.4 GBq (90)Y-DOTATOC. J Nucl Med 2002;43(5):610–6.

105. Grozinsky-Glasberg S, Barak D, Fraenkel M, et al. Peptide receptor radioligand therapy is an effective treatment for the long-term stabilization of malignant gastrinomas. Cancer 2011;117(7):1377–85.

106. Imhof A, Brunner P, Marincek N, et al. Response, survival, and long-term toxicity after therapy with the radiolabeled somatostatin analogue [90Y-DOTA]-TOC in metastasized neuroendocrine cancers. J Clin Oncol 2011;29(17):2416–23.

107. Horsch D, Ezziddin S, Haug A, et al. Effectiveness and side-effects of peptide receptor radionuclide therapy for neuroendocrine neoplasms in Germany: a multi-institutional registry study with prospective follow-up. Eur J Cancer 2016;58:41–51.

108. Strosberg J, El-Haddad G, Wolin E, et al. Phase 3 trial of 177Lu-dotatate for midgut neuroendocrine tumors. N Engl J Med 2017;376(2):125–35.

Precision Medicine and PET–Computed Tomography in Pediatric Malignancies

Yasemin Sanli, MD[a,b],*, Ebru Yilmaz, MD[a],
Rathan M. Subramaniam, MD, PhD, MPH[b,c,d,e,f]

KEYWORDS

• Pediatric malignancies • PET • PET/CT

KEY POINTS

• In Hodgkin lymphoma (HL) and non-Hodgkin lymphoma, fluorine-18 fluorodeoxyglucose (^{18}F-FDG) PET–computed tomography (CT) is the standard of care due to its higher sensitivity in comparison with CT in detecting nodal and extranodal lesions, including lesions in the spleen and bone marrow. In patients with HL, interim ^{18}F-FDG PET/CT is highly sensitive and specific for predicting survival. Multiple trials investigating the role of ^{18}F-FDG PET/CT response-adapted therapy, are ongoing.

• In neuroblastoma, ^{18}F-FDG PET/CT has been found to be superior to CT in detecting distant lymph node metastasis and to bone scintigraphy in detecting skeletal metastasis. Likewise, FDG PET/CT has significantly superior diagnostic ability to that of iodine-131 metaiodobenzylguanidine (^{131}I-MIBG) scintigraphy, especially for the detection of lymph nodal and bone lesions.

• ^{18}F-FDG PET/CT should be part of a standard diagnostic algorithm for children diagnosed with sarcomas, instead of bone imaging with technetium methylene diphosphonate (^{99m}Tc-MDP). Likewise, PET/CT was found to be superior to conventional imaging for detection of lymph node involvement.

• Some evidence in the literature showed correlation between initial standard uptake value (SUV) and histologic differentiation in Wilms tumor. Furthermore, PET/CT may be useful in predicting the response to neoadjuvant chemotherapy in children with Wilms tumor.

INTRODUCTION

More than 12,000 cases of cancers are diagnosed in children in the United States.[1] Cancer is the second most common cause of death among children between the ages of 1 and 14 years. Leukemia (particularly acute lymphocytic leukemia) is the most common cancer in children, followed by cancer of the brain and other nervous system, neuroblastoma (NB), Wilms tumor (WT), and non-Hodgkin lymphoma (NHL).[2] Accurate staging of

Disclosure Statement: None.
[a] Department of Nuclear Medicine, Medical Faculty of Istanbul, Istanbul University, Sehremini, Istanbul 34370, Turkey; [b] Department of Radiology, The University of Texas Southwestern Medical Center, 5323 Harry Hines Boulevard, Dallas, TX 75390-8896, USA; [c] Department of Clinical Sciences, The University of Texas Southwestern Medical Center, 5323 Harry Hines Boulevard, Dallas, TX 75390-8896, USA; [d] Department of Biomedical Engineering, The University of Texas Southwestern Medical Center, 5323 Harry Hines Boulevard, Dallas, TX 75390-8896, USA; [e] Advanced Imaging Research Center, The University of Texas Southwestern Medical Center, 5323 Harry Hines Boulevard, Dallas, TX 75390-8896, USA; [f] Harold C. Simmons Comprehensive Cancer Center, The University of Texas Southwestern Medical Center, 5323 Harry Hines Boulevard, Dallas, TX 75390-8896, USA
* Corresponding author. Department of Radiology, The University of Texas Southwestern Medical Center, 5323 Harry Hines Boulevard, Dallas, TX 75390-8896.
E-mail address: yasemin.sanli@UTsouthwestern.edu

malignant tumors in pediatric patients is utmost importance for appropriate cancer treatment. As treatment of children with cancer has improved to procedure cure rates exceeding 80%, imaging technologies available to clinicians and researchers have evolved to include a wide range of modalities.[3]

Precision nuclear medicine seeks to advance existing and emerging tumor-specific targeting strategies to improve diagnostic imaging and quantification of disease burden while enhancing the multimodality therapeutic options for individual patients. This approach has potential to reduce disease recurrence rates and minimize treatment-related toxicities. Precision nuclear medicine practices must enable better lesion detectability and characterization to determine which treatment modality or modalities are best suited to treat an individual's disease.[4] Accurate staging is important at diagnosis for optimizing the treatment strategy and, after therapy, assessment of treatment response and early detection of recurrence are critical to achieving an optimal outcome.

In pediatric patients, recent evidence demonstrated improved sensitivities and specificities for fluorine-18 fluorodeoxyglucose (^{18}F-FDG) PET and computed tomography (PET/CT) compared with all collective standard staging procedures, especially for patients with lymphomas, sarcomas, and head and neck cancers.[5–7] Diagnostic information obtained from ^{18}F-FDG PET scans changed management in 24% of pediatric oncology patients, including those with lymphoma, sarcoma, central nervous system, and plexiform neurofibroma.[8]

Accordingly, this article aims to review the literature on the use of ^{18}F-FDG PET/CT for initial staging and therapy response of malignant tumors in pediatric patients.

PEDIATRIC BONE AND SOFT TISSUE SARCOMAS

Bone and soft tissue sarcomas account for approximately 10% of all childhood malignancies.[9] Established treatment protocols for sarcoma are multimodal and include surgery, neoadjuvant chemotherapy, adjuvant chemotherapy, and radiation therapy.[10] The most common primary malignant bone tumors in children are osteosarcoma and Ewing sarcoma.[11] In these tumors, subtype of cancer, presence of metastasis, location, and the grade of tumor are factors associated with survival. The overall 5-year survival rate for all localized bone and soft tissue sarcomas is 60% to 70%. However, about 20% to 25% of patients present with metastatic disease

or have refractory or recurrent disease, leading to a poor prognosis.[12] Accurate detection of metastases is important for risk stratification and improved outcomes may be obtained with earlier detection of metastatic disease and with accurate detection of local recurrence following therapy.[13]

Approximately 20% to 25% of patients with osteosarcoma and Ewing sarcoma present with radiographically detectable distant metastases (**Fig. 1**).[14,15] Despite that local or regional nodal spread is rare in osteosarcoma and Ewing sarcoma, they have been reported in up to 20% of children who have rhabdomyosarcoma (RMS).[16,17] On the other hand, bone metastases occur in 10% of patients who have RMS and osteosarcoma. These patients require surgical resection of all sites of metastases for any chance of cure. Because Ewing sarcoma is a radiosensitive tumor, radiotherapy can be beneficial in cases of few and well-circumscribed bone or bone marrow (BM) metastases.[18]

In a retrospective study, Walter and colleagues[19] investigated the need for dedicated bone imaging in addition to ^{18}F-FDG PET/CT imaging in pediatric sarcoma patients. The investigators reported that technetium methylene diphosphonate (^{99m}Tc-MDP) scintigraphy had a lower sensitivity of 70% and an accuracy of 82% when compared with 100% for PET/CT. As a result, they conclude that ^{18}F-FDG PET/CT should be a part of standard diagnostic algorithm for children diagnosed with sarcomas, and bone imaging with ^{99m}Tc-MDP may not be necessary. Meanwhile, Quartuccio and colleagues[20] compared the diagnostic performance of ^{18}F-FDG PET/CT and conventional imaging for staging and follow-up of in 64 pediatric osteosarcoma and skeletal Ewing sarcoma subjects with 412 lesions in a retrospective study. PET/CT was available only at follow-up for osteosarcoma subjects, in which it was proved to be more accurate than conventional imaging for the detection of bone lesions (accuracy, 95% for PET/CT vs 67% for CT and 86% for MR imaging). Both PET/CT and MR imaging were more accurate than CT and bone scanning in the follow-up of both sarcomas. Meanwhile, PET/CT tended to perform better during follow-up than at initial staging (accuracy, 85% vs 69%, respectively) in subjects with Ewing sarcoma. Of note, for lung findings, they found that PET/CT was more specific than CT but was less sensitive. In a similar fashion, London and colleagues[6] included 41 children who were diagnosed with osteosarcoma and Ewing sarcoma in their retrospective analysis. They showed that, excluding lung lesions, PET/CT had higher sensitivity and specificity than other conventional

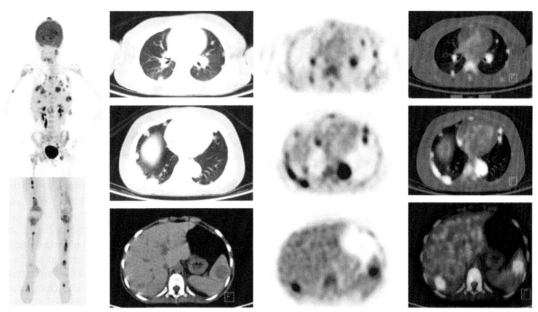

Fig. 1. A 9-year-old girl who had recurrence of primary Ewing sarcoma on left distal femur. Maximum intensity projection images (*right column*) revealed an increased FDG uptake each of the bone metastases. Axial fusion images demonstrated increased FDG uptakes in the bilateral intraparenchymal and subpleural nodules in lungs and bilateral hilar lymph nodes (*first and second rows*), as well as organ metastases in the liver and spleen (*third row*).

imaging such as CT, ultrasound, MR imaging, and/or bone scintigraphy (BS) of 83%, 98%, 78%, 97%, respectively. However, in lung lesions, PET/CT had higher specificity than conventional imaging (96% compared with 87%) but had lower sensitivity (80% compared with 93%). Likewise, Volker and colleagues[21] investigated the value of ^{18}F-FDG PET/CT alone for staging 46 children who had Ewing sarcoma, osteosarcoma, or RMS in their prospective multicenter trial. They found that FDG-PET and conventional imaging modalities were equally effective in the detection of primary tumors (accuracy, 100%). PET was superior to conventional imaging concerning the correct detection of lymph node involvement (sensitivity, 95% vs 25%, respectively) and bone manifestations (sensitivity, 90% vs 57%, respectively), whereas CT was more reliable than FDG-PET in depicting lung metastases (sensitivity, 100% vs 25%, respectively). They showed that 21 of 28 lung metastases detected by CT were missed by FDG-PET and PET-negative nodules were found to be smaller than 7 mm.

Another aspect is that ^{18}F-FDG PET/CT has the potential to provide noninvasive information about necrosis of the primary tumor after chemotherapy and to identify children likely to benefit from further adjuvant therapy before the definitive surgery. Denecke and colleagues[22] reported that overall tumor maximum standard uptake value (SUV$_{max}$) on post-treatment ^{18}F-FDG PET/CT

scans were more accurate for the assessment of therapy response than changes in tumor volume in osteosarcoma subjects. Meanwhile, London and colleagues[6] showed in their study that change in tumor size on MR imaging did not predict response to chemotherapy. In addition, higher initial SUV$_{max}$ and greater SUV$_{max}$ reduction on PET/CT after chemotherapy predicted a favorable response even better than did MR imaging. Also, both PET/CT and MR imaging were very sensitive but of low specificity in predicting physeal tumor involvement. A recent meta-analysis evaluated the predictive value of ^{18}F-FDG PET/CT in the assessment of histologic response to neoadjuvant chemotherapy in subjects with osteosarcomas. Eight studies comprising 178 subjects met the inclusion criteria and it was reported that SUV 2 less than or equal to 2.5 and SUV 2:1 less than or equal to 0.5 were valuable predictors to assess the chemotherapy-induced tumor necrosis.[23]

Despite significant improvements in chemotherapy, approximately 25% to 35% of children and adolescents who have sarcomas experience tumor recurrence after treatment. For this reason, patients are followed clinically and radiographically for 3 to 5 years after therapy and ^{18}F-FDG PET/CT plays the major role in their management.[16,17]

RMS is the most common soft-tissue sarcoma in patients less than 20 years old (60% of soft tissue sarcomas), accounting for approximately 5%

of all pediatric cancers. The 2 main histologic subtypes of RMS tumors are alveolar RMS (ARMS) and embryonal RMS (ERMS). Fibrosarcomas, synovial sarcomas, and extraosseous Ewing sarcomas are the other soft-tissue sarcomas in the pediatric population.[24–26] The major risk factors to predict outcome in RMS are age of the patient, tumor size and invasiveness, primary site and grossly complete surgical removal of localized tumor, existence of alveolar or embryonal differentiation, and presence or absence of metastatic involvement.[27] Approximately 80% of ARMS harbor the reciprocal chromosomal translocation t (2;13) (q35;q14) or the less common variant translocation t (1;13) (p36;q14) in which PAX3 and FOXO1, or PAX7 and FOXO1 genes, respectively, are juxtaposed.[28]

Several studies evaluated the role of PET in the diagnosis, staging, outcome prediction, and monitoring of disease remission and recurrence in subjects with RMS. These studies concluded that ^{18}F-FDG PET/CT provides important additional information in the initial staging of RMS, not only for lymph nodes and metastasis evaluation but also therapeutic management.[29,30] Generally, higher initial SUV_{max} and greater SUV_{max} reduction on PET/CT after chemotherapy predicted a favorable response even better than MR imaging. Federico and colleagues[31] reported the sensitivity, specificity, and accuracy of PET/CT in their retrospective study involving 30 subjects as 94%, 100%, and 95%, respectively, for the detection of lymph node metastases. Meanwhile, another study comprising 35 subjects revealed that PET/CT could correctly diagnose the overall tumor-node-metastasis (TNM) stage in 86% of subjects compared with 54% for conventional imaging modalities such as BS, chest radiograph, CT, or MR imaging ($P<.01$). In addition, PET/CT showed higher accuracies for nodal staging (97% vs 87%) and identifying metastasis (89% vs 63%) in comparison with the conventional imaging.[32] Furthermore, Eugene and colleagues[33] reported in the retrospective evaluation of their 23 RMS subjects that after 3 cycles of chemotherapy ^{18}F-FDG PET/CT found to have 92% of objective response versus 84% for conventional imaging modalities. Meanwhile, Casey and colleagues[34] showed in their retrospective cohort of 107 RMS subjects that baseline PET, PET after induction chemotherapy, and PET after local therapy were all predictive of progression-free survival. Consequently, despite the limited number of studies comprising small numbers of subjects, FDG PET/CT is the preferred imaging modality in RMS for initial staging and evaluation of therapeutic response.

LYMPHOMAS

Lymphomas are the third most common malignancy in the pediatric population and make up approximately 10% to 15% of childhood malignancies. Hodgkin disease (HD) represents 40% of the pediatric lymphomas; whereas NHL represents 60% of the patients.[35] Classic HL accounts for more than 85% of cases of HL and nodular lymphocyte-predominant HL is a less common subtype. NHL tends to be more extranodal compared with HL and shows a predilection for male and white patients.[36] Meanwhile, children generally present with high-grade NHL types such as Burkitt lymphoma, lymphoblastic lymphoma, diffuse large B-cell lymphoma, and anaplastic large cell lymphoma. It should be noted that indolent types of lymphoma seen in adults do not occur in pediatric patients and these subtypes generally show little or no ^{18}F-FDG uptake and usually are not referred for ^{18}F-FDG PET/CT staging examinations.[37,38] Lymphoma is highly curable, with a 5-year overall survival (OS) rate in pediatrics of greater than 90%.[39] In the last decade, some evidence accumulated to show the value of ^{18}F-FDG PET/CT in staging and monitoring treatment response in patients with both HL and NHL.[40] Recently, the staging system of NHL was revised to facilitate more precise staging for children and adolescents with NHL. A similar attempt is also underway for childhood, adolescent, and young adult HL.[41]

Initial Staging

The major advantage of ^{18}F-FDG PET/CT is that it evaluates the functional status of hypermetabolic tissues relatively independent of tumor size.[42] The sensitivities and specificities of ^{18}F-FDG PET/CT for initial staging of malignant lymphomas are 98.7% to 99.2% and 97.6% to 100%, respectively.[43–45] ^{18}F-FDG PET is more sensitive than CT in detecting nodal and extranodal lesions in HL and NHL, including lesions in the spleen and BM (**Fig. 2**).[46,47] Because criteria for disease involvement are usually based on the lesion size and involvement when using morphologic techniques, normal-sized lymph nodes can be missed. In a study by Cheng and colleagues,[39] nodal lesion analyses were performed to assess the performance of ^{18}F-FDG PET/CT versus diagnostic contrast CT in detecting each lymphoma type's involved lymph node or node groups. They showed that PET/CT identified more lesions than diagnostic contrast CT for both subjects with HD and those with NHL in their retrospectively designed study. For subjects with HD, PET/CT and diagnostic contrast CT scans were concordantly positive in 120

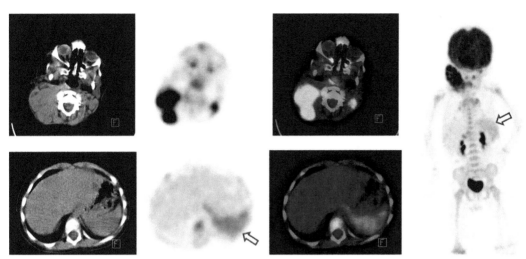

Fig. 2. Baseline PET/CT image of a 3-year-old boy diagnosed with mixed cellularity classic HL who had involvement of cervical lymph nodes and spleen, which upstaged from stage 2 to 3 (*arrows*).

lesions (77.4%). PET/CT detected 94.8% of all lesions, in contrast to 82.6% for diagnostic contrast CT in subjects with HD (*P* = .007). For subjects with NHL, PET/CT and diagnostic contrast CT were concordant in 54 (57.4%) lesions. PET/CT detected 88.3% of all lesions, whereas diagnostic contrast CT detected 69.1% of all lesions (*P* = .013). On the lymph node lesion-based analysis, PET/CT accurately detected 94.8% sites of involvement in HD and detected 88.3% sites of involvement in NHL. In contrast, diagnostic contrast CT detected 82.6% lesions in HD and 69.1% in NHL. Similarly, ^{18}F-FDG PET/CT also identified more extranodal lesions than CT scan in subjects with HD and NHL, especially for BM lesions. Meanwhile, a prospective study comparing ^{18}F-FDG PET with conventional staging methods for initial staging of 55 children and adolescents with HD or NHL revealed that ^{18}F-FDG PET identified 34% additional lesions that were negative on conventional imaging techniques, whereas conventional imaging techniques revealed only 5% additional lesions that were negative on PET. The sensitivity, specificity, and accuracy rates were 96.5% versus 87.5%, 100% versus 60%, and 96.7% versus 85.2% for PET/CT and conventional imaging techniques, respectively.

It should be mentioned that lung metastasis evaluation is the weakest aspect of PET/CT. In a study by Kabickova and colleagues,[46] thoracic CT was reported to be more sensitive than ^{18}F-FDG PET in the detection of pulmonary lesions in HL subjects (100% vs 70%). This is because of the limited spatial resolution of PET by the positron range of ^{18}F-FDG PET, which impairs the detection of small pulmonary nodules and continuous breathing during PET data acquisition.[46,47]

BM involvement is a relatively common feature of advanced NHL, although CT is not sensitive to detect BM involvement (**Fig. 3**). Detection of extranodal lesions such as BM involvement are utmost importance because these extranodal involvement sites upstages the patient to stage IV disease, leading to changes in prognosis and management. For decades, BM biopsy (BMB) has been performed to assess BM infiltration in the initial staging of lymphoma and is considered a gold standard. However, BMB as most commonly taken in the region of the anterior or posterior iliac crests is a relatively invasive procedure and is limited to sampling of only a fraction of the entire BM. In a recent study, Cheng and colleagues[48] reported in pediatric patients that the overall sensitivities of detecting BM involvement by lymphoma was 92% and 54% (*P*<0.05) for ^{18}F-FDG PET and BMB, respectively. Consequently, determination of extranodular lesions, such as BM and spleen, with PET/CT is the standard of care in naïve lymphoma patients.

Therapy Response

The standard therapy of pediatric lymphoma typically involves chemotherapy, which might be followed by the radiotherapy of the disease area in selected cases. Patients with early-stage HL often do not receive radiotherapy, whereas those with intermediate and advanced stages, especially with bulky disease, have improved progression-free survival with the addition of radiotherapy. The criteria for the definition of adequate or inadequate response in children with HL are still under discussion.[49] The International Harmonization Project first published guidelines about the application of PET

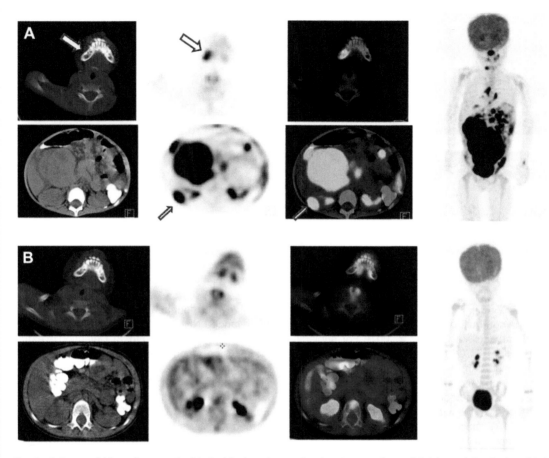

Fig. 3. A 3-year-old boy diagnosed with Burkitt lymphoma. Staging images showed (*A*) intraabdominal multiple lymph nodes and conglomerate mass, bone involvement of the right mandibular (*thick arrows*) and right kidney involvement (*thin arrow*). In therapy, response imaging (*B*) showed complete anatomic and metabolic response.

using ^{18}F-FDG in lymphoma in 2007 by Juweid and colleagues[50] and revised by Cheson and colleagues.[51] In 2009, at the First International Workshop in France, on interim-PET in lymphoma, a 5-point scoring scale (Deauville criteria), for visual evaluation of interim PET-scans were proposed, which is currently considered the international standard.[52] In practice, an interim FDG-PET scan after 1 or 2 cycles of chemotherapy is basically used to evaluate treatment and tailor adapted therapy in malignant lymphoma.[53–55] The rational of this approach is to identify patients with an inadequate response and determine the patients who could benefit from treatment intensification. On the contrary, treatment burden can be reduced in PET-negative patients because it is particularly important to avoid therapy-related sequelae and secondary malignancies in children and adolescents with HL.[56–58] In patients with HL, interim FDG-PET/CT is highly sensitive and specific for predicting survival, and multiple trials to study FDG-PET/CT response-adapted therapy are

ongoing. Furth and colleagues[59] reported in a prospective study with 40 HL subjects that a negative interim ^{18}F-FDG PET/CT scan after 2 cycles of chemotherapy is a strong indicator of relapse-free survival, with a negative predictive value of 100%. On the other hand, Bakhshi and colleagues[60] compared the use of interim or post-treatment PET/CT using Deauville criteria to predict clinical outcome, as well as event-free survival and OS. And also they compared these results between PET/CT and contrast-enhanced CT (CECT) in pediatric HL subjects. They showed that specificity of interim PET/CT with Deauville criteria for predicting relapse was higher than CECT; 91.4% versus 40.3%, respectively. Specificity of post-treatment PET/CT with Deauville criteria for predicting relapse was 95.7% versus 76.4% by CECT. They showed that in the evaluation of the OS between subjects who were positive or negative by post-treatment PET/CT with Deauville criteria, a significant difference was detected in favor of poor survival (66.4 ± 22.5 vs 94.5 ± 2.0, respectively;

P = .029). The event-free survival did not differ in subjects who were positive or negative based on interim or post-treatment PET/CT response with Deauville criteria. In their multicentric retrospective design study with 165 early stage HL subjects, Ciammella and colleagues[61] suggested that ^{18}F-FDG PET at the end of chemotherapy was a strong prognostic marker, especially for subjects with interim ^{18}F-FDG PET positivity. They showed that when combining the interim and end of chemotherapy ^{18}F-FDG PET results, the 5-year PFS were 97%, 100%, and 82% in negative-negative, positive-negative, and positive-positive groups, respectively. Although interim FDG-PET/CT is highly sensitive and specific for predicting survival in patients with HL, results of ^{18}F-FDG PET/CT are not widely used to guide therapy in patients with NHL. This is primarily because of the heterogeneity of tumor and lack of evidence of a reasonable positive predictive value.[62–64] Bakhshi and colleagues[65] recruited 34 subjects with nonlymphoblastic NHL in prospective study. They reported that PET/CT may be better than CECT for routine baseline investigation. Briefly, PET/CT findings upstaged the disease in 5 (14.7%) subjects, demonstrated 18 additional disease sites in 15 subjects that were found to be statistically significant. In addition, 100% (4 subjects) concordance was observed between BM involvement at biopsy and stage at PET/CT. After a mean follow-up of 20.3 months, interim PET/CT and CECT findings were not found to be predictive for PFS and OS. In addition, post-treatment PET/CT and CECT findings could predict PFS and post-treatment CECT findings could predict OS; however, post-treatment PET/CT findings could not predict OS.

Technological advancements have made possible to detect the related genes that contribute to disease pathogenesis and evolution, especially in major lymphoma subtypes. A recent review article identified MYD88, BRAF, ID3, TCF3, STAT3, STAT5B, RHOA, TET2, and IDH2 mutations are the only genes that can be considered as a complement to the current set-up for lymphoma diagnostics.[66] In the pathogenesis of lymphomas, the most important mechanism of MYC overexpression is constituted by chromosomal rearrangements leading to repositioning of MYC under the control of a potent enhancer like those of the immunoglobulins. In Burkitt lymphoma, MYC rearrangements are considered as the hallmark of this disease and a translocation is found in almost all cases.[67] Meanwhile, in a recent study, La Nasa and colleagues[68] evaluated the correlation of killer immunoglobulin-like receptor (KIR) genes and KIR haplotypes with the achievement of interim PET/CT in a cohort of 135 subjects

(age range: 8–60 years) with advanced stage classic HL. The investigators reported that homozygosity for KIRA haplotype was present with a significantly higher frequency in subjects with negative interim PET/CT (36.3% vs 15.2%, P = .03) after 2 cycles of chemotherapy. Meanwhile, homozygosity for KIR A haplotype remained the only predictive factor for the achievement of negative interim PET/CT in the multivariate analysis.

NEUROBLASTOMA

NB is the most common extracranial solid cancer in childhood. It is also among the leading causes of cancer-related death in children. Half of the NBs arise from the adrenal glands. Other common sites are the neck, chest, and pelvis. They particularly occur in children, with a median age at diagnosis of 17 months. Approximately 70% of patients have distant metastasis, and the most common sites of metastasis are bone and BM, at the time of diagnosis.[69–73]

NB cells have the unique capacity to accumulate iodine (I)-123 metaiodobenzylguanidine (^{123}I-MIBG), which can be used for single-photon emission computed tomography (SPECT) imaging the primary tumor and metastases. Meanwhile, ^{131}I-MIBG is also used for targeted radionuclide therapy with positive ^{123}I-MIBG scan. However, ^{123}I-MIBG scan has some limitations that should be taken into consideration. Approximately, 10% of NBs do not show MIBG uptake. Furthermore, medications such as phenylephrine, labetalol, and tricyclic antidepressants may alter the MIBG biodistribution. In these patients, bone scans and [18]FDG PET scans were useful additional tools for whole-body staging.[74,75] In a prospective study, Papathanasiou and colleagues[76] performed both FDG PET and ^{123}I-MIBG scintigraphy in 28 subjects with refractory or relapsed high-risk NB. The investigators found that tumoral FDG uptake and the FDG skeletal extent score were significant prognostic factors for OS in contrast to the ^{123}I-MIBG skeletal score. However, it should be noted that FDG PET has limitations in detecting bone or BM metastasis because it demonstrates increased uptake of ^{18}F-FDG due to BM hyperplasia after myelosuppressive chemotherapy, particularly in advanced stages of NB. Meanwhile, Dhull and colleagues[77] and Choi and colleagues[78] showed significantly superior diagnostic ability of ^{18}F-FDG PET/CT to that of ^{131}I-MIBG scintigraphy, especially for the detection of lymph nodal and bone lesions. Dhull and colleagues[77] investigated 28 subjects undergoing both imaging studies. The sensitivity, specificity, positive-predictive value, negative-predictive value, and accuracy of ^{18}F-FDG PET/CT were 100%, 60%, 92%, 100%, and 92.8%, respectively. For ^{131}I-MIBG, they were 95.6%, 60%, 91.6%, 75%, and 89.2%, respectively. Meanwhile, in the study by Choi and colleagues,[78] who recruited 30 subjects with pathologically proven NB, diagnostic performance of ^{18}F-FDG PET and abdomen CT were compared in detecting soft tissue lesions. In addition, FDG PET and BS were compared for bone metastases. FDG PET was found to be superior to CT in detecting distant lymph node metastasis and to BS in detecting skeletal metastasis. Thus, the investigators concluded that BS might be eliminated in the evaluation of NB when ^{18}F-FDG PET is performed. High-resolution images can be acquired with FDG-PET/CT with excellent anatomic delineation (**Fig. 4**). Another advantage of ^{18}F-FDG-PET scan

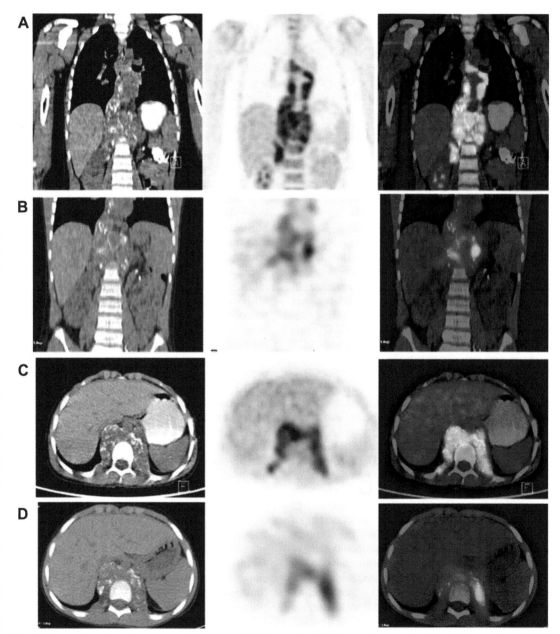

Fig. 4. Restaging of a primary neuroblastoma with FDG PET/CT (*A* [coronal images] – *C* [axial images]) and ^{123}I-MIBG (*B* [coronal images] – *D* [axial images]) at the time of relapse 1 year after initial therapy of an 11-year-old boy. Both studies demonstrated thoracic and abdominal conglomerate lymph nodes, which moderately increased ^{123}I-MIBG uptake and highly increased FDG-avid lesions.

is the lack of need for thyroid blockade, as well as the withholding of drugs.

New radiotracers such as [124]I-metaiodobenzyl-guanidine ([124]I-MIBG PET), ^{18}F-dihydroxyphenyla-lanine (^{18}F-DOPA), and ^{18}F-MIBG may be the future for NB staging and treatment monitoring.[79–81] These tracers may enable theranostic approaches with combined diagnostic and therapeutic tracers. Kroiss and colleagues[82] analyzed ^{68}Ga-DOTA-Tyr[3]-octreotide (^{68}Ga-DOTA-TOC) PET/CT in a small cohort of subjects, providing particularly valu-able information for pretherapeutic staging of NB that may be superior to ^{123}I-MIBG imaging. In this study, the sensitivity of ^{68}Ga-DOTA-TOC for NB was 97.2% and for ^{123}I-MIBG was 90.7%.

High-risk NB patients are characterized by age, stage, and histopathology, as well as MYCN amplification.[72] The study by Liu and colleagues[83] revealed that subjects with older age, advanced stages, or MYCN amplification showed higher FDG and lower ^{18}F-DOPA SUV_{max} values. Receiver operating characteristics analysis identi-fied FDG SUV_{max} equal to or greater than 3.31 and ^{18}F-DOPA SUV_{max} less than 4.12 as an ultra-high-risk feature that distinguished the most unfavor-able genomic types, such as segmental chromo-somal alterations and/or MYCN amplification, at a sensitivity of 81.3% and a specificity of 93.3%. Higher glycolytic activity and less catecholamin-ergic differentiation in NB tumors taking up higher FDG and lower ^{18}F-DOPA was an independent predictor of inferior event-free survival in consider-ation with age, stage, MYCN status, and anatomic image-defined risk factor. Meanwhile, it was also mentioned that intensity of ^{18}F-FDG and ^{18}F-DOPA uptake on diagnostic PET scans may predict the tumor behavior and complement the current risk stratification systems of NB.

WILMS TUMOR

Among the pediatric solid tumors, WT is the second most common, accounting for 6% of all pediatric cancer in the United States.[84] At diag-nosis, the mean age of patients at diagnosis is approximately 3.5 years, and 75% are younger than 5 years.[85] With modern combined therapeutic strategies, such as chemotherapy, radiotherapy, and surgery, overall long-term survival is more than 90%.[86] Despite this good prognosis, higher stage disease carries significant mortality and treatment-related morbidities. Meanwhile, it was shown that chromosomal abnormalities, such as gain of 1q (1q+) is increasingly being proposed as a common prognostic biomarker to select pa-tients for more intensive treatment.[87] In addition, loss of heterozygosity of chromosomes 1p and

16q revealed high-risk histologic features and not independent adverse prognostic factors.[88]

Tumor location and size, local extension, vascular compression or invasion, and local lymph node metastases are important issues for staging that are best evaluated with conventional imaging techniques. These techniques rely on the docu-mentation of morphologic changes, and have limited accuracy and reproducibility in determining clinical downstaging and distinguishing viable tu-mor from fibrotic tissue.[89] However, the role of FDG-PET in WT has not been well established and limited articles exist in this topic. Misch and colleagues[90] evaluated 23 ^{18}F-FDG-PET scans of 12 subjects with WT for staging and found a good correlation between initial SUV and histolog-ic differentiation. Of the 12 subjects, 6 underwent ^{18}F-FDG-PET scanning before and after neoadju-vant chemotherapy for preoperative response assessment. PET parameters failed to reveal a reli-able indicator for therapy success in their study with respect to local control or progression-free survival. Meanwhile, Qin and colleagues[89] recruited 12 subjects who underwent PET/CT. Five had nonmetastatic at diagnosis and 7 sub-jects had metastasis at diagnosis. The histologic subtype was intermediate in 10 subjects and anaplastic in 2 subjects. They showed a good correlation of changes in SUV_{max} and pathologic response, and they stated that PET/CT has the po-tential of predicting the response to neoadjuvant chemotherapy in children with WT.

PET/MR IMAGING

Radiation exposure in children may cause more serious consequences than in adults. The risk of radiation-induced cancer mortality is significantly higher per unit dose in children than in adults because this risk increases inversely with age.[91] ^{18}F-FDG PET/MR imaging has an obvious advan-tage over PET/CT in the form of radiation dose reduction, as much as 45%, because of the lack of ionizing radiation. The ability to perform func-tional imaging, multiparametric imaging, and the use of soft tissue contrast are the other advan-tages of PET/MR imaging. Sher and colleagues[92] compared the diagnostic performance of ^{18}F-FDG PET/MR imaging with that of ^{18}F-FDG PET/CT in a cohort of pediatric lymphoma subjects. They observed no statistical difference between the 2 modalities in terms of lesion detection and the accuracy of staging. Quantification of ^{18}F-FDG uptake using SUV measurements showed that there was a strong correlation between PET/CT and PET/MR imaging but that SUVs were underestimated by PET/MR imaging. Moreover, the investigators showed that sequential PET/MR imaging is comparable to the data obtained with PET/CT in terms of lesion detection. They compared with the reference standard and found there was no significant difference in lesion classification between PET/MR imaging and PET/CT for sensitivity (92% vs 95%, respectively; $P = 1$) or specificity (61% vs 56%; $P = 1$). Both PET/MR imaging and PET/CT showed an overall classification accuracy of 82%. In a similar study, Ponisio and colleagues[93] demonstrated an average percent radiation exposure reduction of 39% plus or minus 13% with PET/MR imaging compared with PET/CT. Moreover, they showed that PET/MR imaging performance was comparable to PET/CT for lesion detection and SUV measurements. However, it should be noted that both studies had insufficient number of subjects (25 and 8) and further studies with extended numbers of subjects are needed to determine the exact value of PET/MR in pediatric lymphomas.

REFERENCES

1. Cancer incidence and survival among children and adolescents: United States SEER Program 1975-1995. Bethesda (MD): National Cancer Institute, SEER Program. NIH Pub. No. 99-4649; 1999.
2. Padma S, Sundaram PS, Tewari A. PET/CT in paediatric malignancies - an update. Indian J Med Paediatr Oncol 2016;37:131–40.
3. Weiser DA, Kaste SC, Siegel MJ, et al. Imaging in childhood cancer: a Society for Pediatric Radiology and Children's Oncology Group joint task force report. Pediatr Blood Cancer 2013;60:1253–60.
4. Wright CL, Maly JJ, Zhang J, et al. Advancing precision nuclear medicine and molecular imaging for lymphoma. PET Clin 2017;12:63–82.
5. Baum SH, Frühwald M, Rahbar K, et al. Contribution of PET/CT to prediction of outcome in children and young adults with rhabdomyosarcoma. J Nucl Med 2011;52:1535–40.
6. London K, Stege C, Cross S, et al. 18F-FDG PET/CT compared to conventional imaging modalities in pediatric primary bone tumors. Pediatr Radiol 2012;42:418–30.
7. Boktor RR, Omar WS, Mousa E, et al. A preliminary report on the impact of 18F-FDG PET/CT in the management of paediatric head and neck cancer. Nucl Med Commun 2012;33:21–8.
8. Wegner EA, Barrington SF, Kingston JE, et al. The impact of PET scanning on management of paediatric oncology patients. Eur J Nucl Med Mol Imaging 2005;32:23–30.
9. Amankwah EK, Conley AP, Reed DR. Epidemiology and therapies for metastatic sarcoma. Clin Epidemiol 2013;5:147–62.
10. Parida L, Fernandez-Pineda I, Uffman J, et al. Clinical management of Ewing sarcoma of the bones of the hands and feet: a retrospective single- institution review. J Pediatr Surg 2012;47:1806–10.
11. Kaste SC. Imaging pediatric bone sarcomas. Radiol Clin North Am 2011;49:749–65.
12. Krishnan K, Khanna C, Helman LJ. The biology of metastases in pediatric sarcomas. Cancer J 2005; 11:306–13.
13. Potter DA, Glenn J, Kinsella T, et al. Patterns of recurrence in patients with high-grade soft-tissue sarcomas. J Clin Oncol 1985;3:353–66.
14. Marina N, Gebhardt M, Teot L, et al. Biology and therapeutic advances for pediatric osteosarcoma. Oncologist 2004;9:422–41.
15. Quartuccio N, Cistaro A. Primary bone tumors. In: Cistara A, editor. Atlas of PET/CT in pediatric patients. Heidelberg (Germany): Springer; 2014.
16. Link MP, Gebhardt M, Meyers P. Osteosarcoma. In: Pizzo P, Poplack D, editors. Principles and practice of pediatric oncology. 5th edition. Philadelphia: Lippincott Williams & Wilkins; 2006. p. 1074–115.
17. Bernstein M, Kovar H, Paulussen M, et al. Ewing sarcoma family of tumors: Ewing sarcoma of bone and soft tissue and the peripheral primitive neuroectodermal tumors. In: Pizzo P, Poplack D, editors. Principles and practice of pediatric oncology. 5th edition. Philadelphia: Lippincott, Williams & Wilkins; 2006. p. 1002–32.
18. McCarville MB. PET and PET/CT in pediatric sarcomas. PET Clin 2008;3:563–75.
19. Walter F, Czernin J, Hall T, et al. Is there a need for dedicated bone imaging in addition to 18F-FDG PET/CT imaging in pediatric sarcoma patients. J Pediatr Hematol Oncol 2012;34:131–6.
20. Quartuccio N, Fox J, Kuk D, et al. Pediatric bone sarcoma: diagnostic performance of 18F-FDG PET/CT versus conventional imaging for initial staging and follow-up. AJR Am J Roentgenol 2015;204:153–60.
21. Volker T, Denecke T, Steffen I, et al. Positron emission tomography for staging of pediatric sarcoma patients: results of a prospective multicenter trial. J Clin Oncol 2007;25:5435–41.
22. Denecke T, Hundsdörfer P, Misch D, et al. Assessment of histological response of paediatric bone sarcomas using FDG PET in comparison to morphological volume measurement and standardized MRI parameters. Eur J Nucl Med Mol Imaging 2010;37:1842–53.
23. Hongtao L, Hui Z, Bingshun W, et al. 18F-FDG positron emission tomography for the assessment of histological response to neoadjuvant chemotherapy in osteosarcomas: a meta-analysis. Surg Oncol 2012; 21:e165–70.
24. Ognjanovic S, Linabery AM, Charbonneau B, et al. Trends in childhood rhabdomyosarcoma incidence and survival in the United States, 1975-2005. Cancer 2009;115:4218–26.

25. Arndt CA, Crist WM. Common musculoskeletal tumors of childhood and adolescence. N Engl J Med 1999;341:342–52.

26. Paulino AC, Okcu MF. Rhabdomyosarcoma. Curr Probl Cancer 2008;32:7–34.

27. Raney RB, Anderson JR, Barr FG, et al. Rhabdomyosarcoma and undifferentiated sarcoma in the first two decades of life: a selective review of intergroup rhabdomyosarcoma study group experience and rationale for Intergroup Rhabdomyosarcoma Study V. J Pediatr Hematol Oncol 2001;23:215–20.

28. Parham DM, Barr FG. Classification of rhabdomyosarcoma and its molecular basis. Adv Anat Pathol 2013;20:387–97.

29. McLean TW, Buckley KS. Pediatric genitourinary tumors. Curr Opin Oncol 2010;22:268–73.

30. Roberge D, Vakilian S, Alabed YZ, et al. FDG PET/CT in initial staging of adult soft-tissue sarcoma. Sarcoma 2012;2012:960194.

31. Federico SM, Spunt SL, Krasin MJ, et al. Comparison of PET-CT and conventional imaging in staging pediatric rhabdomyosarcoma. Pediatr Blood Cancer 2013;60:1128–34.

32. Tateishi U, Hosono A, Makimoto A, et al. Comparative study of FDG PET/CT and conventional imaging in the staging of rhabdomyosarcoma. Ann Nucl Med 2009;23:155–61.

33. Eugene T, Corradini N, Carlier T, et al. F-18 FDG PET/CT in initial staging and assessment of early response to chemotherapy of pediatric rhabdomyosarcomas. Nucl Med Commun 2012;33:1089–95.

34. Casey DL, Wexler LH, Fox JJ, et al. Predicting outcome in patients with rhabdomyosarcoma: role of [(18)f]fluorodeoxyglucose positron emission tomography. Int J Radiat Oncol Biol Phys 2014;1(90):1136–42.

35. Depas G, De Barsy C, Jerusalem G, et al. 18F-FDG PET in children with lymphomas. Eur J Nucl Med Mol Imaging 2005;32:31–8.

36. Percy CL, Smith MA, Linet M, et al. Lymphomas and reticuloendothelial neoplasms. In: Ries LAG, Smith MA, Gurney JG, et al, editors. Cancer incidence and survival among children and adolescents:United States SEER Program. Bethesda (MD): NIH; 1999. p. 35–50.

37. Chung EM, Pavio M. Pediatric Extranodal Lymphoma. Radiol Clin North Am 2016;54:727–46.

38. Burton C, Ell P, Linch D. The role of PET imaging in lymphoma. Br J Haematol 2004;126:772–84.

39. Cheng G, Servaes S, Alavi A, et al. FDG PET and PET/CT in the management of pediatric lymphoma patients. PET Clin 2008;3:621–34.

40. Rosolen A, Perkins SL, Pinkerton CR, et al. Revised international pediatric non-Hodgkin lymphoma staging system. J Clin Oncol 2015;33:2112–8.

41. Flerlage JE, Kelly KM, Beishuizen A, et al. Staging evaluation and response criteria harmonization

(SEARCH) for childhood, adolescent and young adult Hodgkin lymphoma (CAYAHL): methodology statement. Pediatr Blood Cancer 2017. http://dx.doi.org/10.1002/pbc.26421.

42. Kumar R, Maillard I, Schuster SJ, et al. Utility of fluorodeoxyglucose-PET imaging in the management of patients with Hodgkin, and non-Hodgkin's lymphomas. Radiol Clin North Am 2004;42:1083–100.

43. Miller E, Metser U, Avrahami G, et al. Role of 18F-FDG PET/CT in staging and follow-up of lymphoma in pediatric and young adult patients. J Comput Assist Tomogr 2006;30:689–94.

44. Paulino AC, Margolin J, Dreyer Z, et al. Impact of PET-CT on involved field radiotherapy design for pediatric Hodgkin lymphoma. Pediatr Blood Cancer 2012;58:860–4.

45. Punwani S, Taylor SA, Bainbridge A, et al. Pediatric and adolescent lymphoma: comparison of whole-body STIR half-Fourier RARE MR imaging with an enhanced PET/CT reference for initial staging. Radiology 2010;255:182–90.

46. Kabickova E, Sumerauer D, Cumlivska E, et al. Comparison of 18F-FDG-PET and standard procedures for the pretreatment staging of children and adolescents with Hodgkin's disease. Eur J Nucl Med Mol Imaging 2006;33:1025–31.

47. Cheng G, Servaes S, Zhuang H. Value of 18F-fluoro-2-deoxy-D-glucose positron emission tomography/computed tomography scan versus diagnostic contrast computed tomography in initial staging of pediatric patients with lymphoma. Leuk Lymphoma 2013;54:737–42.

48. Cheng G, Chen W, Chamroonrat W, et al. Biopsy versus FDG PET/CT in the initial evaluation of bone marrow involvement in pediatric lymphoma patients. Eur J Nucl Med Mol Imaging 2011;38:1469–76.

49. Hasenclever D, Kurch L, Mauz-Körholz C, et al. qPET - a quantitative extension of the Deauville scale to assess response in interim FDG-PET scans in lymphoma. Eur J Nucl Med Mol Imaging 2014;41:1301–8.

50. Juweid ME, Stroobants S, Hoekstra OS, et al. Use of positron emission tomography for response assessment of lymphoma: consensus of the Imaging Subcommittee of International Harmonization Project in Lymphoma. J ClinOncol 2007;25:571–8.

51. Cheson BD, Pfistner B, Juweid ME, et al. Revised response criteria for malignant lymphoma. J ClinOncol 2007;25:579–86.

52. Meignan M, Gallamini A, Meignan M, et al. Report on the first international Workshop on interim-PET-scan in lymphoma. Leuk Lymphoma 2009;50:1257–60.

53. Engert A, Haverkamp H, Kobe C, et al. Reduced-intensity chemotherapy and PET-guided radiotherapy in patients with advanced stage Hodgkin's lymphoma (HD 15 trial): a randomised, open-label,

phase 3 non-inferiority trial. Lancet 2012;379: 1791–9.

54. Gonzalez-Barca E, Canales M, Cortes M, et al. Predictive value of interim 18F-FDG-PET/CT for event free survival in patient with diffuse large B-cell lymphoma homogenously treated in a phase II trial with six cycles of R-CHOP-14 plus pegfilgrastim as first line treatment. Nucl Med Commun 2013;34: 946–52.

55. Gallamini A, Patti C, Viviani S, et al. Early chemotherapy intensification with BEACOPP in advanced-stage Hodgkin lymphoma patients with an interim–PET positive after two ABVD courses. Br J Haematol 2011;152:551–60.

56. Schellong G, Riepenhausen M, Bruch C, et al. Late valvular and other cardiac diseases after different doses of mediastinal radiotherapy for Hodgkin disease in children and adolescents: report from the longitudinal GPOH follow-up project of the German-Austrian DAL-HD studies. Pediatr Blood Cancer 2010;1(55):1145–52.

57. Kostakoglu L, Gallamini A. Interim 18F-FDG PET in Hodgkin lymphoma: would PET-adapted clinical trials lead to paradigm shift? J Nucl Med 2013;54: 1082–93.

58. Gallamini A, Rigacci L, Merli F, et al. The predictive value of positron emission tomography scanning performer after two courses of standard therapy on treatment outcome in advanced stage Hodgkin's disease. Haematologica 2006;91:475–81.

59. Furth C, Steffen IG, Amthauer H, et al. Early and late therapy response assessment with [18F] fluorodeoxyglucose positron emission tomography in pediatric Hodgkin's lymphoma: analysis of a prospective multicenter trial. J ClinOncol 2009;10(27):4385–91.

60. Bakhshi S, Bhethanabhotla S, Kumar R, et al. Posttreatment PET-CT rather than interim PET-CT using Deauville criteria predicts outcome in pediatric Hodgkin lymphoma: a prospective study comparing PET-CT versus conventional imaging. J Nucl Med 2016;58:577–83.

61. Ciammella P, Filippi AR, Simontacchi G, et al. Post-ABVD/pre-radiotherapy (18)F-FDG-PET provides additional prognostic information for early-stage Hodgkin lymphoma: a retrospective analysis on 165 patients. Br J Radiol 2016;89:20150983.

62. Moskowitz CH, Schoder H, Teruya-Feldstein J, et al. Risk-adapted dose-dense immunochemotherapy determined by interim FDG-PET in Advanced-stage diffuse large B-Cell lymphoma. J Clin Oncol 2010;28:1896–903.

63. Moskowitz CH, Zelenetz A, Schoder H. An update on the role of interim restaging FDG-PET in patients with diffuse large B-cell lymphoma and Hodgkin lymphoma. J Natl Compr Canc Netw 2010;8:347–52.

64. Terasawa T, Lau J, Bardet S, et al. Fluorine-18-fluorodeoxyglucose positron emission tomography for interim response assessment of advanced-stage Hodgkin's lymphoma and diffuse large B-cell lymphoma: a systematic review. J Clin Oncol 2009;27: 1906–14.

65. Bakhshi S, Radhakrishnan V, Sharma P, et al. Pediatric nonlymphoblastic non-Hodgkin lymphoma: baseline, interim, and posttreatment PET/CT versus contrast-enhanced CT for evaluation-a prospective study. Radiology 2012;262:956–68.

66. Rosenquist R, Rosenwalt A, Du MQ, et al. Clinical impact of recurrently mutated genes on lymphoma diagnostics: state-of-the-art and beyond. Haematologica 2016;101:1002–9.

67. Haberl S, Haferlach T, Stengel A. MYC rearranged B-cell neoplasms: impact of genetics on classification. Cancer Genet 2016;209:431–9.

68. La Nasa G, Greco M, Littera R, et al. The favorable role of homozygosity for killer immunoglobulin-like receptor (KIR) A haplotype in patients with advanced-stage classic Hodgkin lymphoma. J Hematol Oncol 2016;16:9–26.

69. DuBois SG, Kalika Y, Lukens JN, et al. Metastatic sites in stage IV and IVS neuroblastoma correlate with age, tumor biology, and survival. J Pediatr Hematol Oncol 1999;21:181–9.

70. Matthay KK, Villablanca JG, Seeger RC, et al. Treatment of high-risk neuroblastoma with intensive chemotherapy, radiotherapy, autologous bone marrow transplantation, and 13-cis-retinoic acid. Children's Cancer Group. N Engl J Med 1999;341: 1165–73.

71. Maris JM, Hogarty MD, Bagatell R, et al. Neuroblastoma. Lancet 2007;369:2106–20.

72. Maris JM. Recent advances in neuroblastoma. N Engl J Med 2010;362:2202–11.

73. Park JR, Eggert A, Caron H. Neuroblastoma: biology, prognosis, and treatment. Pediatr Clin North Am 2008;55:97–120.

74. Sharp SE, Gelfand MJ, Shulkin BL. Pediatrics: diagnosis of neuroblastoma. Semin Nucl Med 2011;41: 345–53.

75. Piccardo A, Lopci E, Conte M, et al. PET/CT imaging in neuroblastoma. Q J Nucl Med Mol Imaging 2013; 57:29–39.

76. Papathanasiou ND, Gaze MN, Sullivan K, et al. 18F-FDG PET/CT and 123I-metaiodobenzylguanidine imaging in high-risk neuroblastoma: diagnostic comparison and survival analysis. J Nucl Med 2011;52: 519–25.

77. Dhull VS, Sharma P, Patel C, et al. Diagnostic value of 18F-FDG PET/CT in paediatric neuroblastoma: comparison with 131I-MIBG scintigraphy. Nucl Med Commun 2015;36:1007–13.

78. Choi YJ, Hwang HS, Kim HJ, et al. (18)F-FDG PET as a single imaging modality in pediatric neuroblastoma: comparison with abdomen CT and bone scintigraphy. Ann Nucl Med 2014;28:304–13.

79. Vaidyanathan G, Affleck DJ, Zalutsky MR. Validation of 4-[fluorine-18]fluoro-3-iodobenzylguanidine as a positron-emitting analog of MIBG. J Nucl Med 1995;36:644–50.

80. Lopci E, Piccardo A, Nanni C, et al. 18F-DOPA PET/CT in neuroblastoma: comparison of conventional imaging with CT/MR. Clin Nucl Med 2012;37:73–8.

81. Zhang H, Huang R, Pillarsetty N, et al. Synthesis and evaluation of 18F-labeledbenzylguanidine analogs for targeting the human norepinephrine transporter. Eur J Nucl Med Mol Imaging 2014;41:322–32.

82. Kroiss A, Putzer D, Uprimny C, et al. Functional imaging in phaeochromocytoma and neuroblastoma with 68Ga-DOTA-Tyr3-octreotide positron emission tomography and 123I-metaiodobenzylguanidine. Eur J Nucl Med Mol Imaging 2011;38(5):865–73.

83. Liu YL, Lu MY, Chang HH, et al. Diagnostic FDG and FDOPA positron emission tomography scans distinguish the genomic type and treatment outcome of neuroblastoma. Oncotarget 2016;5:18774–86.

84. Ries LAG, Eisner MP, Kosary CL, et al. SEER cancer statistics review, 1975–2000. Bethesda (MD): National Cancer Institute; 2003.

85. Dome JS, Perlman EJ, Richey ML, et al. Renal tumors. In: Pizzo PA, Poplack DG, editors. Principles and practice of pediatric oncology. Philadelphia: Lippincott Williams & Wilkins; 2006. p. 905–32.

86. Mitchell C, Jones PM, Kelsey A, et al. The treatment of Wilms' tumour: results of the United Kingdom Children's Cancer Study Group (UKCCSG) second Wilms' tumour study. Br J Cancer 2000;83:602–8.

87. Segers H, van den Heuvel-Eibrink MM, Williams RD, et al. Gain of 1q is a marker of poor prognosis in Wilms' tumors. Children's Cancer and Leukaemia Group and the UK Cancer Cytogenetics Group. Genes Chromosomes Cancer 2013;52:1065–74.

88. Sredni ST, Gadd S, Huang CC, et al. Subsets of very low risk Wilms tumor show distinctive gene expression, histologic, and clinical features. Clin Cancer Res 2009;15:6800–9.

89. Qin Z, Tang Y, Wang H, et al. Use of 18F-FDG-PET-CT for assessment of response to neoadjuvant chemotherapy in children with Wilms tumor. J Pediatr Hematol Oncol 2015;37:396–401.

90. Misch D, Steffen IG, Schönberger S, et al. Use of positron emission tomography for staging, preoperative response assessment and posttherapeutic evaluation in children with Wilms tumour. Eur J Nucl Med Mol Imaging 2008;35:642–50.

91. NRC. Health risks from exposure to low levels of ionizing radiation: BEIR VII phase 2. Washington, DC: The National Academies Press; 2006. p. 269–71.

92. Sher AC, Seghers V, Paldino MJ, et al. Assessment of sequential PET/MRI in comparison with PET/CT of pediatric lymphoma: a prospective study. AJR Am J Roentgenol 2016;206:623–31.

93. Ponisio MR, McConathy J, Laforest R, et al. Evaluation of diagnostic performance of whole-body simultaneous PET/MRI in pediatric lymphoma. Pediatr Radiol 2016;46:1258–68.

PET/Computed Tomography and Precision Medicine: Gastric Cancer

Charles Marcus, MD[a,b,]*,
Rathan M. Subramaniam, MD, PhD, MPH[a,c,d,e,f,g]

KEYWORDS

- Gastric cancer • Gastric carcinoma • Gastric lymphoma • PET • PET/CT

KEY POINTS

- National Comprehensive Cancer Network guidelines for the management of gastric cancer workup algorithm for patients with newly diagnosed gastric cancer includes fluorine-18 fluoro-2-deoxy-D-glucose PET/computed tomography (^{18}F-FDG PET/CT) evaluation, especially when metastatic cancer is not evident and in the use of ^{18}F-FDG PET/CT in the posttreatment assessment and restaging of these patients.
- The metabolic activity of the primary tumor in the staging ^{18}F-FDG PET/CT may help in surgical planning and identifying different gastric cancer histopathologies.
- ^{18}F-FDG PET/CT provides value in detecting metastases, especially distant metastases and synchronous second malignancies, treatment response assessment and modifying therapy for individual patients.
- ^{18}F-FDG PET/CT has good performance in the detection or recurrent disease and follow-up of these patients.
- The metabolic tumor markers measured in an ^{18}F-FDG PET/CT study can provide valuable prognostic information.

INTRODUCTION

There are about 7.4 new cases of gastric cancer per 100,000 men and women per year in the United States. It is the fifteenth leading cause of cancer death. The number of deaths estimated is 3.3 per 100,000 men and women per year, between 2009 and 2013. The lifetime risk of developing gastric cancer is approximately 0.9%. The estimated number of new cases in 2016 is 26,370, and the estimated number of deaths due

Disclosure Statement: None.
[a] The Russell H. Morgan Department of Radiology and Radiological Sciences, The Johns Hopkins University School of Medicine, 601 North Caroline Street, Baltimore, MD 21287, USA; [b] Department of Nuclear Medicine, Johns Hopkins Medical Institutions, JHOC 3224, Baltimore, MD 21287, USA; [c] Department of Radiology, The University of Texas Southwestern Medical Center, 5323 Harry Hines Boulevard, Dallas, TX 75390-8896, USA; [d] Department of Clinical Sciences, The University of Texas Southwestern Medical Center, Harry Hines Boulevard, Dallas, TX 75390, USA; [e] Department of Biomedical Engineering, The University of Texas Southwestern Medical Center, Harry Hines Boulevard, Dallas, TX 75390, USA; [f] Department of Nuclear Medicine, Advanced Imaging Research Center, The University of Texas Southwestern Medical Center, Harry Hines Boulevard, Dallas, TX 75390, USA; [g] Department of Nuclear Medicine, Harold C. Simmons Comprehensive Cancer Center, The University of Texas Southwestern Medical Center, Harry Hines Boulevard, Dallas, TX 75390, USA
* Corresponding author. Department of Nuclear Medicine, Johns Hopkins Medical Institutions, JHOC 3224, Baltimore, MD 21287.
E-mail address: cmarcus7@jhmi.edu

PET Clin 12 (2017) 437–447
http://dx.doi.org/10.1016/j.cpet.2017.05.004
1556-8598/17/© 2017 Elsevier Inc. All rights reserved.

to gastric cancer is 10,730. Gastric cancer is more common in men than women and other ethnicities than non-Hispanic whites. Age, diet, and stomach disease, including infection with *Helicobacter pylori*, can affect the risk of developing gastric cancer. The overall 5-year survival for gastric cancer is only 30.4%. The 5-year survival decreases with the stage of the disease, ranging from 66.9% in patients with localized disease to 30.9% in regional disease and 5.0% in distant disease, respectively.[1] The treatment algorithm of gastric cancer ranges from surgical resection to palliative systemic therapy depending on the clinical stage of the disease and warrants accurate staging of the disease and appropriate treatment planning to improve the survival in these patients. Imaging plays a vital role in accurate and rapid staging of these patients. According to the National Comprehensive Cancer Network (NCCN) guidelines for the management of gastric cancer, the workup algorithm for patients with newly diagnosed gastric cancer includes fluorine-18 fluoro-2-deoxy-D-glucose PET/computed tomography (^{18}F-FDG PET/CT) evaluation, if clinically indicated and if metastatic cancer is not evident. It also recommends the use of ^{18}F-FDG PET/CT in the post-treatment assessment and restaging of these patients.[2] The histopathology of gastric tumors varies depending on which layer of the stomach they arise from. Most gastric cancers arise from the glands of the gastric mucosa and are classified as adenocarcinomas. Gastric cancers can also originate from other components of the stomach, such as the lymphoid tissue, neuroendocrine cells, or the muscular layers of the stomach wall. The behavior of gastric tumors varies based on their histopathology, and hence, the treatment plan is also tailored to the type of gastric cancer.[3,4]

Although most gastric cancers have been found to be sporadic, true hereditary gastric cancers contribute to a very small proportion of patients. It has been found that nearly 40% of hereditary gastric cancers exhibit mutated CDH1, leading to defective or loss of expression of E-cadherin, which in turn results in activation of epidermal growth factor receptor (EGFR). Genetic susceptibility to gastric cancer may also be conferred by several single nucleotide polymorphisms, particularly in the genes coding for inflammatory cytokines, such as interleukin-1, tumor necrosis factor-α, and so forth, and carbone metabolism methylenetetrahydrofolate reductase, which play a critical role in regulation of DNA methylation and epigenetic modulation. Several signaling pathways are known to be altered during gastric carcinogenesis, and the precise cause-and-effect relationship for these

changes is not clear. The altered pathways include EGFR, c-MET oncogene overexpression, vascular endothelial growth factor receptor, mammalian target of rapamycin, fibroblast growth factor, Hedgehog PATCH1 smoothened pathway, mitogen-activated protein kinase, and kinase-extracellular signal-regulated kinase pathway. Many of these altered pathways are involved in cell proliferation, angiogenesis, apoptosis, and cell cycle and can result in cancer. An important target in human malignancy is the EGFR family. This family includes EGFR/HER1, HER2/neu, HER3, and HER4. Stimulation of pathways involving these receptors influences cell proliferation, differentiation, migration, and apoptosis. HER2/new oncogene amplification results in HER2-receptor overexpression and can enhance and prolong signals that lead to uncontrolled cell growth and tumorigenesis. The incidence of HER2-positive gastric cancer has been reported to be as high as 22%. These targets are also being used for directed therapies.[5–7]

^{18}F-FDG PET/CT has been shown to provide valuable information in the staging, treatment response evaluation, detecting recurrence, follow-up, and prognosis in patients with gastric cancer. Some studies have also shown that the imaging of gastric cancers is also possible with the proliferation marker [18]F Fluorothymidine, and that it can be more sensitive in gastric tumors without or with low FDG activity. It has also shown good performance in the evaluation of the primary tumor and regional lymph nodes.[8–10] The aim of this review article is to provide a concise summary of the available literature on ^{18}F-FDG PET/CT and its role in the evaluation and management of gastric cancer.

DIAGNOSIS AND STAGING OF GASTRIC CANCER

The role of ^{18}F-FDG PET/CT in the evaluation of the primary tumor, locoregional and distant lymph node involvement, and distant metastases has been described in the following few sections. The final importance of these findings is that ^{18}F-FDG PET/CT plays an important role in accurately staging these patients and thereby having an impact on the management and prognosis of these patients: tailoring the therapy for these patients and influencing the outcomes. In a study involving 608 patients with biopsy-proven gastric adenocarcinoma, FDG-PET changed the stage in 28.9% patients. Of those who were upstaged, 64.5% developed progressive disease.[11] Similarly, in gastric lymphoma, ^{18}F-FDG PET/CT changed the stage in up to 35% of patients with a primary gastric lymphoma.[12]

EVALUATION OF THE PRIMARY TUMOR

Multiple studies have shown that ^{18}F-FDG PET/CT may not contribute significantly toward the evaluation of the primary gastric tumor. Altini and colleagues[11] demonstrated that there was no significant difference in either sensitivity or specificity between the widely used contrast-enhanced computed tomography (CECT) and ^{18}F-FDG PET/CT for the evaluation of the primary gastric lesion. Although primary tumor evaluation by ^{18}F-FDG PET/CT has not gained much importance, it may provide additional information that may be of use to the treating clinician. In a study by Hur and colleagues[13] in 2010, the investigators concluded that the level of FDG uptake may predict noncurative resection in patients with advanced gastric cancer. The level of FDG uptake in the primary tumor may provide valuable information to the operating surgeon. In their study, Hur and colleagues[13] demonstrated that the primary tumor mean standardized uptake value (SUV) of patients who underwent noncurable operations was significantly higher than that of patients with curable surgeries ($P = .001$). Positive FDG uptake in primary tumors ($P = .047$) and local lymph nodes ($P<.001$) was related to noncurable operations. The correlation between the level of FDG uptake and noncurable surgeries may help treating clinicians decide on other treatment modalities without surgery. Factors such as age, tumor depth, tumor size, lymph node metastases, and clinical stage of the disease and the presence of distant metastases seem to play a role in the findings seen in patients with gastric cancer, undergoing an ^{18}F-FDG PET/CT study. Oh and colleagues[14] showed that the primary tumor peak-SUV was associated with age ($P = .009$), tumor depth ($P<.001$), tumor size ($P<.001$), and lymph node metastases ($P<.001$). They demonstrated that a higher peak-SUV was associated with lymph node metastases. Namikawa and colleagues[15] demonstrated this by showing that the median maximum standardized uptake value (SUV$_{max}$) was significantly higher in patients with T3/T4 tumors in comparison to T1/T2 tumors (9.0 versus 3.8; $P<.001$) in patients with distant metastasis than in those with no metastasis (9.5 versus 7.7; $P = .018$) and in stage 3/4 disease than in stage 1/2 disease (9.0 versus 4.7; $P = .017$). The SUV$_{max}$ of the primary tumor was significantly correlated with tumor size ($P<.001$). In the recent past, human epidermal growth factor receptor 2 (HER2) expression in gastric cancer has gained importance, with studies demonstrating that HER2-targeted molecular therapies are highly relevant in the treatment of gastric cancer. Chen and colleagues[12] evaluated ^{18}F-FDG PET/CT as a potential noninvasive strategy for predicting the mutation profile in patients with gastric cancers and found that there may be some relationship between the tumor SUV$_{max}$ and tumor differentiation with HER2 expression. They also demonstrated that the SUV$_{max}$ was significantly higher in HER2-negative patients, when signet-ring-cell carcinoma was excluded, in their study involving 64 patients with gastric cancer. The FDG avidity of a tumor is known to be positively correlated to the tumor proliferation. Deng and colleagues[16] evaluated the correlation between the tumor FDG uptake and the antigen Ki-67, which is a well-known tumor proliferation marker in patients with cancer. The investigators performed a meta-analysis including 79 articles (n = 3242) and found that the FDG uptake showed that the correlation between FDG uptake and Ki-67 expression was significant in gastrointestinal stromal tumors (GIST) in their subgroup analysis. They report a correlation coefficient of 0.72 (95% confidence interval 0.58–0.85; $P<.05$) in the 4 studies on GISTs. In routine clinical practice, a relatively common interpretation dilemma is differentiating benign gastric lesions from gastric cancer in patients with focally increased gastric uptake. In recent years, dual time point imaging with ^{18}F-FDG PET/CT has been shown to help in this situation. Dual time point imaging done at 1 and 2 hours after radiotracer administration demonstrated that 85% patients with increased SUV$_{max}$ in the delayed imaging had a malignant lesion and 90% patients with decreased SUV$_{max}$ in the delayed imaging had a benign lesion, with statistical significance of the change in SUV$_{max}$ values between the 2 groups ($P = .000$).[17] ^{18}F-FDG PET/CT may also be useful in differentiating gastric tumors based on their histopathology. Although tissue diagnosis is inevitable before treatment, this information may help treating physicians in the accurate diagnosis of these patients. Fu and colleagues[18] demonstrated that patients with aggressive non-Hodgkin lymphoma exhibited a higher SUV$_{max}$, corrected for maximal gastrointestinal wall thickness, than patients with advanced gastric carcinoma ($P<.05$) and mucosa-associated lymphoid tissue (MALT) ($P<.05$). The pattern of FDG uptake may exhibit certain differences that may help differentiate gastric cancer from gastric lymphoma. Three patterns of FDG activity have been described: type I, diffuse thickening of the gastric wall with increased FDG uptake infiltrating more than one-third of the total stomach; type II, segmental thickening of the gastric wall with elevated FDG uptake involving less than one-third of the total stomach; and type III, local thickening of the gastric wall with focal FDG uptake. A study has shown that gastric lymphoma predominantly presented with type I and II lesions, whereas gastric cancer mainly presented in type II and III lesions[19] (Figs. 1 and 2). However, Radan and colleagues[20] noticed FDG avidity in 89% of primary gastric lymphoma, including all patients with aggressive non-Hodgkin's lymphoma, but only 71% of MALT. However, the investigators found that the intensity of FDG activity, rather than the pattern, was more useful in differentiating primary gastric lymphoma from normal stomach. They found an SUV_{max} of 15.3 ± 11.7 in primary gastric lymphoma as opposed to 4.6 ± 1.4 in controls (P<.001). In patients with advanced gastric cancer, a commonly observed finding is that the ^{18}F-FDG avidity of primary signet-ring-cell carcinoma and mucinous adenocarcinoma was

significantly lower than that of other types of adenocarcinomas, such as well-differentiated, moderately differentiated, or poorly differentiated tubular adenocarcinomas, papillary adenocarcinomas, and so forth (Fig. 3). Kawanaka and colleagues[21] found that the mean SUV_{max} values between these 2 groups were 6.43 ± 3.48 versus 8.95 ± 5.73, (P = .015). Yi and colleagues[22] have shown that in patients with primary gastric lymphoma, SUV_{max} above median value in their study population was significantly associated with an advanced Lugano stage (P<.001). There is limited literature on other gastric cancer histopathologies. Case reports on gastric sarcomas have described the pattern of FDG uptake in these lesions as intense peripheral uptake with central photopenia within ill-defined heterogeneous masses.[23] A small study (n = 29) of GISTs, with the most common site being stomach (41.0%), showed that ^{18}F-FDG PET/CT was useful in

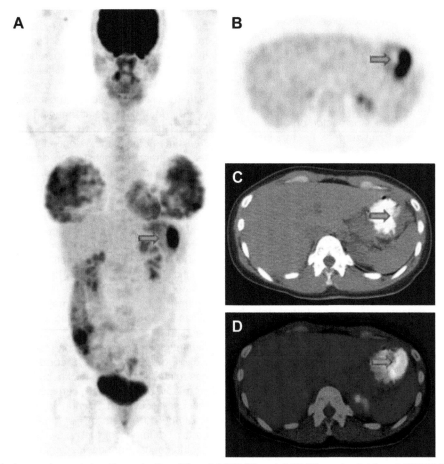

Fig. 1. Anterior maximum intensity projection (A), axial PET (B), axial CT (C), and axial fused PET/CT (D) images from a staging ^{18}F-FDG PET/CT of a 39-year-old woman with a recently diagnosed invasive poorly differentiated carcinoma of the stomach demonstrating an intensely hypermetabolic (SUV_{max} 10.34) gastric wall thickening (blue arrows) in the body, antrum, and greater curvature of the stomach, consistent with the primary lesion. Symmetric physiologic radiotracer uptake is noted in the breast tissue.

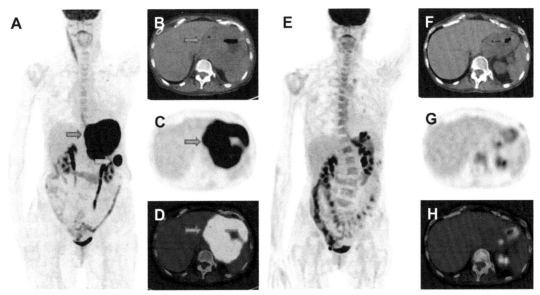

Fig. 2. Anterior maximum intensity projection (*A*), axial CT (*B*), axial PET (*C*), and axial fused PET/CT (*D*) images from a staging ^{18}F-FDG PET/CT of a 69-year-old woman who had a gastrointestinal bleed and was diagnosed with a large gastric mass. Biopsy of the lesion showed diffuse large B-cell lymphoma. The PET/CT images demonstrate a diffusely and intensely FDG-avid (SUV$_{max}$ 17.9) large multilobular mass involving the walls of the stomach (*blue arrows*). The images also demonstrate an FDG-avid peritoneal implant (*yellow arrow*). The anterior maximum intensity projection (*E*), axial CT (*F*), axial PET (*G*), and axial fused PET/CT (*H*) images from the restaging ^{18}F-FDG PET/CT after 2 cycles of chemotherapy demonstrate interval reduction in thickening and FDG activity in the gastric wall, compatible with treatment response.

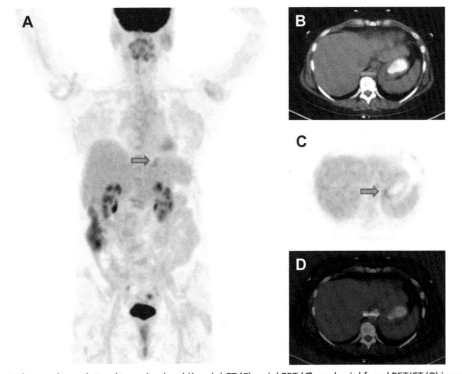

Fig. 3. Anterior maximum intensity projection (*A*), axial CT (*B*), axial PET (*C*), and axial fused PET/CT (*D*) images from a staging ^{18}F-FDG PET/CT of a 43-year-old woman who was diagnosed with gastric cancer and underwent a total gastrectomy. Surgical pathology revealed signet-ring-cell carcinoma. The PET/CT shows mildly increased FDG activity (SUV$_{max}$ 2.12) (*blue arrows*) in the stomach wall corresponding to the wall thickening noted on the CT study.

determining the extent of the disease in patients treated with imatinib.[24]

EVALUATION OF LYMPH NODE AND DISTANT METASTASIS

Although ^{18}F-FDG PET/CT may not have a role in detection of the primary gastric tumor, it plays an important role in the detection of lymph node metastasis, especially distant lymph node involvement and distant metastasis.[25] ^{18}F-FDG PET/CT may have a higher specificity and positive predictive value in the detection of lymph node metastases than CECT. In comparison to the performance of the widely used CECT, a study by Altini and colleagues[11] on 45 patients with a newly diagnosed gastric cancer before treatment demonstrated that specificity of ^{18}F-FDG PET/CT was significantly higher in comparison to CECT for both lymph node and distant metastasis (95.24% versus 61.9%; 88.57% versus 62.86%, respectively). However, there has been some controversy on this topic, with some clinicians stating that ^{18}F-FDG PET/CT may not be accurate in preoperative staging of gastric cancer because of its low sensitivity in predicting lymph node metastasis.[26] On the other hand, studies have shown that the sensitivity, specificity, and accuracy of ^{18}F-FDG PET/CT are not significantly different for N2 and N3 disease and that the high specificity of PET for lymph node disease may be clinically valuable and presence of N disease on PET may have a clinically significant impact on the choice of therapy.[27] In a recent study of 106 patients with advanced gastric cancer, Kawanaka and colleagues[21] compared CECT and ^{18}F-FDG PET/CT and showed that the patient-based sensitivity, specificity, and accuracy for the detection of distant lymph node metastases were significantly better for ^{18}F-FDG PET/CT and CECT combination than CECT alone (P = .013, .0077, and .049, respectively). However, the investigators did not find any statistically significant difference between the 2 modalities for the diagnosis of regional lymph node metastasis, peritoneal dissemination, liver metastasis, metastasis at other sites, or overall distant metastasis. The histology of the primary gastric tumor may play a role in the detection of lymph node metastases. Signet-ring-cell histology has shown to trend toward non-FDG-avid lymph node metastases (odds ratio = 0.15, P = .093).[28] A summary of the diagnostic accuracies of ^{18}F-FDG PET/CT and CECT in the detection of lymph node metastases has been presented in **Table 1**.

To overcome the unsatisfactory detection rates in primary tumors and regional metastatic lymph nodes often secondary to small lesions or due to high background FDG activity in the gastric wall, certain imaging techniques have been evaluated. Lee and colleagues[29] found that the sensitivity for both primary tumor (P<.005) and regional lymph node metastasis (P<.01) was significantly improved by regional PET/CT over gastric area

Table 1
Diagnostic accuracy of fluorine-18 fluoro-2-deoxy-ᴅ-glucose PET/computed tomography and contrast-enhanced computed tomography in the evaluation of lymph node metastases from gastric cancer

Study	Modality	Sensitivity, %	Specificity, %	Positive Predictive Value, %	Negative Predictive Value, %	Accuracy, %
Yang et al,[52] 2008	CT	60.5	83.3	82.1	62.5	70.6
	PET/CT	31.0	97.2	92.9	54.7	61.5
Kim et al,[37,53] 2011	CECT	75.0	92.0	98.0	42.0	77.0
Regional LN metastases	PET/CT	41.0	100.0	100.0	26.0	51.0
Namikawa et al,[15] 2014	PET/CT	64.5	85.7	90.9	52.2	71.1
Park et al,[28] 2014 Regional	CECT	51.0	79.0	—	—	64.0
LN metastases	PET/CT	34.0	88.0	—	—	58.0
Filik et al,[54] 2015	CECT	83.3	75.0	87.5	66.6	80.0
	PET/CT	64.7	100.0	100.0	57.1	76.0
Altini et al,[11] 2015	CECT	70.83	61.90	68.0	65.0	66.66
	PET/CT	58.33	95.24	93.33	66.67	75.55
Kawanaka et al,[21] 2016	CECT	45.9	98.0	—	—	75.6
Distant LN metastases	PET/CT + CECT	67.6	100.0	—	—	86.0
Kawanaka et al,[21] 2016	CECT	84.0	70.0	—	—	82.4
Regional LN metastases	PET/CT + CECT	80.0	70.0	—	—	78.8

performed 80 minutes after radiotracer administration after water gastric inflation, whereas the specificity of the whole-body PET/CT was not compromised by regional PET/CT. A prospective study (n = 113) evaluating the role of ^{18}F-FDG PET/CT in staging locally advanced gastric cancer showed that it detected occult metastatic disease in 10% of patients. Economic modeling suggested that the addition of ^{18}F-FDG PET/CT to the standard staging evaluation of these patients resulted in an estimated cost savings of ~USD 13,000 per patient[30] (see **Fig. 2**). In patients with bone metastases from gastric cancer, ^{18}F-FDG PET/CT may be effective for the diagnosis of bone metastases in the initial staging workup. Ma and colleagues[31] reviewed the studies of 170 patients with suspected bone metastasis, of whom 81.2% were confirmed to have bone metastasis, and found that the sensitivity, specificity, positive predictive value, negative predictive value, and accuracy of ^{18}F-FDG PET/CT and whole-body bone scintigraphy were 93.5%, 25.0%, 84.3%, 47.1%, 80.6% and 93.5%, 37.5%, 86.6%, 57.1%, 82.9%, respectively. They also showed that 15.0% of solitary metastases were positive on ^{18}F-FDG PET/CT only. The investigators concluded that ^{18}F-FDG PET/CT may be superior to bone scintigraphy for the detection of synchronous bone metastasis, but the 2 modalities were similar in the detection of metachronous bone metastasis.

DETECTION OF SYNCHRONOUS PRIMARY CANCERS

^{18}F-FDG PET/CT is beneficial in patients with a possible synchronous second malignancy, because it not only evaluates the stage of the primary gastric cancer but can also screen for synchronous tumors because it allows evaluation of the whole body in one sitting. Studies have shown that patients with gastric cancer may be at an increased risk of a synchronous colorectal cancer. Choi and colleagues[32] evaluated 256 patients who underwent colonoscopy and ^{18}F-FDG PET/CT and showed that ^{18}F-FDG PET/CT demonstrated a high diagnostic accuracy (94.5%) in detecting a synchronous colorectal cancer in 4.7% of their study population.

EVALUATION OF TREATMENT RESPONSE

The metabolic changes in tumors in comparison to the baseline study before treatment can be evaluated by ^{18}F-FDG PET/CT and can be a valuable indicator of systemic therapy response that can guide further management in these patients. The

available literature evaluating this in gastric cancers is limited. Couper and colleagues[33] evaluated 14 patients with esophageal (n = 2) and gastric cancer (n = 12) who underwent chemotherapy. Thirteen of these patients had a baseline ^{18}F-FDG PET/CT study before treatment for comparison. A change in the tumor-to-liver ratio was seen in all 13 patients (median reduction 22%), ranging from complete response to 15% increase. These findings were also correlated with anatomic changes in CT imaging and patient symptoms. For example, in 6 patients with more than 30% reduction in the tumor-to-liver ratio, 4 had a partial response detected on CT. The findings were also correlated with the quality of life of these patients in terms of symptoms such as dysphagia, weight loss/gain, and so forth, and these patients had shown either no change or improvement in their symptoms. They also showed that the shortest survival was seen in a patient with increased tumor-to-liver ratio after chemotherapy (see **Fig. 2**).

DETECTION OF DISEASE RECURRENCE AND FOLLOW-UP

^{18}F-FDG PET/CT may have a role in the detection and evaluation of gastric cancer recurrence with moderate sensitivity and specificity, especially in FDG-avid primary tumors, which then results in appropriate change in management and thus outcome in these patients. A recent study by Kim and colleagues[34] of 368 patients with advanced gastric cancer who underwent ^{18}F-FDG PET/CT for initial staging and for recurrence surveillance after curative surgery showed that of the 19.6% of patients who had recurrence, the sensitivity was higher in scans of patients with FDG-avid than nonavid tumors (81.0% versus 52.4%; P = .018) and nonanastomosis site recurrences (82.1% versus 47.45; P = .006). A similar trend was also seen for detecting peritoneal recurrence. The PET specificity for these 2 groups was 97.1% and 97.5%, respectively. A meta-analysis of 8 studies including 500 patients evaluating the value of ^{18}F-FDG PET/CT for the detection of gastric cancer recurrence after surgical resection showed a sensitivity, specificity, positive likelihood ratio, and negative likelihood ratio of 86.0%, 88.0%, 17.0, and 0.16, respectively.[35] In another meta-analysis by Wu and colleagues[36] of 9 studies (n = 526), the investigators found that the sensitivity and specificity for ^{18}F-FDG PET in detecting recurrent gastric cancer was 0.72 and 0.84, respectively. The corresponding values for CECT were 0.74 and 0.85, respectively. The values for combined PET and CT were 0.75 and 0.85, respectively. The investigators suggested that

^{18}F-FDG PET combined with CT can improve the detection rates of recurrent gastric cancer. In a study by Kim and colleagues[37] on 139 patients, the investigators found no statistical significance in the sensitivity, specificity, or accuracy between PET/CT and CECT in detecting tumor recurrence after curative resection, except in the detection of peritoneal carcinomatosis, which was statistically significant (P = .021). However, PET/CT had detected a second malignancy in 8 patients (colon cancer, n = 4; thyroid cancer, n = 3; prostate cancer, n = 1). Similar advantage of PET/CT in diagnosing a second malignancy was observed by Nakamoto and colleagues,[38] and superior performance of CECT in detecting peritoneal metastases was reported by Sim and colleagues.[39] The FDG uptake of the primary tumor at baseline appears to be able to predict subsequent recurrence. Lee and colleagues[40] found that the 24-month recurrence-free survival was significantly higher in patients with negative FDG uptake (95%) than those with a positive FDG uptake (74%) ($P<.0001$). Similar prognostic correlation was only marginally significant in patients with signet-ring-cell carcinoma and mucinous carcinoma (P = .05), in comparison to tubular adenocarcinoma (P = .003) or poorly differentiated adenocarcinoma (P = .0001). Sharma and colleagues,[41] in their study of 72 patients, found that the lesionwise accuracy of ^{18}F-FDG PET/CT in detecting local recurrence was 89.2%, 94.6% for lymph nodes, 96.7% for liver, 96.7% for lung, 98.9% for bone,

and 98.9% for other sites. They found that the accuracy was lower for local recurrence as compared with that of liver (P = .012) and bone (P = .012). However, the number of patients with distant metastases in their study population was low in comparison to local or lymph node metastases and may explain the high accuracies in distant sites. Studies have also shown FDG uptake at the anastomotic site may have to be reported with caution, because most of these have been shown to be false positives, sometimes persisting over several follow-up scans.[42,43] ^{18}F-FDG PET/CT also seems to have good diagnostic ability in postoperative surveillance in patients with gastric cancer.[44] A summary of the diagnostic accuracies of different studies evaluating ^{18}F-FDG PET/CT to detect recurrent gastric cancer disease is presented in **Table 2**.

PREDICTION OF PROGNOSIS

In patients with metastatic gastric adenocarcinoma, a study by Chung and colleagues[45] of 35 newly diagnosed patients showed that a primary tumor SUV$_{max}$ value higher than 8 was a significant independent prognostic predictor of overall survival (P = .048). Similarly, in a study of 321 patients, the investigators found that a primary tumor SUV$_{max}$ higher than 5.74 was a poor prognostic indicator of progression-free survival (P = .034, hazard ratio [HR] 3.59).[46] Another study found that the SUV$_{max}$ of the stomach was an independent

Table 2
Fluorine-18 fluoro-2-deoxy-D-glucose PET/computed tomography in the detection of gastric cancer recurrence

Study	Type of Study	SN	SP	PPV	NPV	Accuracy	PLR	NLR
Park et al,[55] 2009	Retrospective (n = 105)	0.75	0.77	0.89	0.55	0.75	—	—
Nakamoto et al,[38] 2009	Retrospective (n = 92)	0.86	0.94	0.96	0.79	0.89	—	—
Sim et al,[39] 2009	Retrospective (n = 52)	0.68	0.71	0.86	—	—	—	—
Kim et al,[37] 2011	Retrospective (n = 139)	0.54	0.85	—	—	0.78	—	—
Lee et al,[56] 2011	Retrospective (n = 89)	0.43	0.60	0.29	0.78	0.57	—	—
Wu et al,[36] 2012	Meta-analysis of 9 studies (n = 526)	0.78	0.82	—	—	—	3.52	0.32
Sharma et al,[41] 2012		—	—	—	—	—	—	—
Zou et al,[35] 2013	Meta-analysis of 8 studies (n = 500)	0.86	0.88	—	—	—	17.0	0.16
Cayvarli et al,[57] 2014	Retrospective (n = 130)	0.91	0.62	0.85	0.75	0.82	—	—
Lee et al,[42] 2014	Retrospective (n = 46)	1.00	0.88	0.44	1.00	—	—	—
Li et al,[58] 2016	Meta-analysis of 14 studies (n = 828)	0.85	0.78	—	—	—	3.9	0.19

Abbreviations: NLR, negative likelihood ratio; NPV, negative predictive value; PLR, positive likelihood ratio; PPV, positive predictive value; SN, sensitivity; SP, specificity.

predictor of both progression-free survival (*P* = .002) and overall survival (*P* = .038) in patients with metastatic gastric cancer, before treatment.[47] It is known that aggressive tumors have a higher mitotic rate and correlate to higher FDG uptake and poor prognosis. Park and colleagues[48] found significant correlation between the SUV$_{max}$, Ki-67 index, tumor size, and mitotic count in 26 patients with gastric GISTs. In a multivariate regression analysis, Grabinska and colleagues[49] found that metabolic tumor markers like total lesion glycolysis at 30% SUV$_{max}$ threshold was significant for overall survival (HR = 1.001, *P* = .047) and time to metastasis (HR 1.006, *P* = .02) in their study of 40 patients with gastric cancer. In contrast, Na and colleagues[50] found that the primary tumor maximum and peak tumor-to-liver ratios were significantly unfavorable for recurrence-free survival (*P*<.05 for both), and metabolic tumor volume and total lesion glycolysis did not show such trend. The FDG activity in metastatic lymph nodes can also provide prognostic information. Song and colleagues[51] found that the nodal SUV $_{max}$ measured preoperatively was an independent risk factor for both recurrence-free survival (*P*<.0001, HR = 2.71) and overall survival (*P*<.0001, HR = 2.80).

SUMMARY

In ^{18}F-FDG PET/CT, although limited in the evaluation of the primary tumor as such, the metabolic information of primary gastric tumors in an ^{18}F-FDG PET/CT study can assist in surgical and treatment planning and differentiating gastric cancers. It detects nodal disease with good specificity and positive predictive value. It provides valuable information about distant metastases and detecting recurrent disease and in the follow-up of patients. The NCCN workup algorithm for patients with newly diagnosed gastric cancer includes ^{18}F-FDG PET/CT evaluation, especially if metastatic cancer is not evident. It also recommends the use of ^{18}F-FDG PET/CT in the posttreatment assessment and restaging of these patients.

REFERENCES

1. NIH. SEER stat fact sheets: stomach cancer 2011-2013. 2016. Available at: https://seer.cancer.gov/statfacts/html/stomach.html. Accessed January 6, 2017.
2. NCCN. National Comprehensive Cancer Network guidelines: gastric cancer. 2016. Available at: https://www.nccn.org/professionals/physician_gls/pdf/gastric.pdf. Accessed January 6, 2017.
3. Cheng XJ, Lin JC, Tu SP. Etiology and prevention of gastric cancer. Gastrointest Tumors 2016;3(1):25–36.
4. Bordi C. Neuroendocrine pathology of the stomach: the Parma contribution. Endocr Pathol 2014;25(2):171–80.
5. Kelly CM, Janjigian YY. The genomics and therapeutics of HER2-positive gastric cancer-from trastuzumab and beyond. J Gastrointest Oncol 2016;7(5):750–62.
6. Zhang XY, Zhang PY. Gastric cancer: somatic genetics as a guide to therapy. J Med Genet 2017;54(5):305–12.
7. Yuan DD, Zhu ZX, Zhang X, et al. Targeted therapy for gastric cancer: current status and future directions (Review). Oncol Rep 2016;35(3):1245–54.
8. Herrmann K, Ott K, Buck AK, et al. Imaging gastric cancer with PET and the radiotracers 18F-FLT and 18F-FDG: a comparative analysis. J Nucl Med 2007;48(12):1945–50.
9. Staniuk T, Malkowski B, Srutek E, et al. Comparison of FLT-PET/CT and CECT in gastric cancer diagnosis. Abdom Radiol (NY) 2016;41(7):1349–56.
10. Staniuk T, Zegarski W, Malkowski B, et al. Evaluation of FLT-PET/CT usefulness in diagnosis and qualification for surgical treatment of gastric cancer. Contemp Oncol (Pozn) 2013;17(2):165–70.
11. Altini C, Niccoli Asabella A, Di Palo A, et al. 18F-FDG PET/CT role in staging of gastric carcinomas: comparison with conventional contrast enhancement computed tomography. Medicine (Baltimore) 2015;94(20):e864.
12. Chen R, Zhou X, Liu J, et al. Relationship between 18F-FDG PET/CT findings and HER2 expression in gastric cancer. J Nucl Med 2016;57(7):1040–4.
13. Hur H, Kim SH, Kim W, et al. The efficacy of preoperative PET/CT for prediction of curability in surgery for locally advanced gastric carcinoma. World J Surg Oncol 2010;8:86.
14. Oh HH, Lee SE, Choi IS, et al. The peak-standardized uptake value (P-SUV) by preoperative positron emission tomography-computed tomography (PET-CT) is a useful indicator of lymph node metastasis in gastric cancer. J Surg Oncol 2011;104(5):530–3.
15. Namikawa T, Okabayshi T, Nogami M, et al. Assessment of (18)F-fluorodeoxyglucose positron emission tomography combined with computed tomography in the preoperative management of patients with gastric cancer. Int J Clin Oncol 2014;19(4):649–55.
16. Deng SM, Zhang W, Zhang B, et al. Correlation between the uptake of 18F-fluorodeoxyglucose (18F-FDG) and the expression of proliferation-associated antigen Ki-67 in cancer patients: a meta-analysis. PLoS One 2015;10(6):e0129028.
17. Cui J, Zhao P, Ren Z, et al. Evaluation of dual time point imaging 18F-FDG PET/CT in differentiating

malignancy from benign gastric disease. Medicine (Baltimore) 2015;94(33):e1356.

18. Fu L, Li H, Wang H, et al. SUVmax/THKmax as a biomarker for distinguishing advanced gastric carcinoma from primary gastric lymphoma. PLoS One 2012;7(12):e50914.

19. Wu J, Zhu H, Li K, et al. 18F-fluorodeoxyglucose positron emission tomography/computed tomography findings of gastric lymphoma: comparisons with gastric cancer. Oncol Lett 2014;8(4):1757–64.

20. Radan L, Fischer D, Bar-Shalom R, et al. FDG avidity and PET/CT patterns in primary gastric lymphoma. Eur J Nucl Med Mol Imaging 2008;35(8): 1424–30.

21. Kawanaka Y, Kitajima K, Fukushima K, et al. Added value of pretreatment (18)F-FDG PET/CT for staging of advanced gastric cancer: comparison with contrast-enhanced MDCT. Eur J Radiol 2016;85(5): 989–95.

22. Yi JH, Kim SJ, Choi JY, et al. 18F-FDG uptake and its clinical relevance in primary gastric lymphoma. Hematol Oncol 2010;28(2):57–61.

23. Gamble B, Meka M, Ho L. F-18 FDG PET-CT imaging in gastric sarcoma. Clin Nucl Med 2009;34(9): 564–5.

24. Valls-Ferrusola E, Garcia-Garzon JR, Ponce-Lopez A, et al. Patterns of extension of gastrointestinal stromal tumors (GIST) treated with imatinib (Gleevec(R)) by 18F-FDG PET/CT. Rev Esp Enferm Dig 2012;104(7):360–6.

25. Dassen AE, Lips DJ, Hoekstra CJ, et al. FDG-PET has no definite role in preoperative imaging in gastric cancer. Eur J Surg Oncol 2009;35(5):449–55.

26. Ha TK, Choi YY, Song SY, et al. F18-fluorodeoxyglucose-positron emission tomography and computed tomography is not accurate in preoperative staging of gastric cancer. J Korean Surg Soc 2011;81(2): 104–10.

27. Yun M, Lim JS, Noh SH, et al. Lymph node staging of gastric cancer using (18)F-FDG PET: a comparison study with CT. J Nucl Med 2005;46(10):1582–8.

28. Park K, Jang G, Baek S, et al. Usefulness of combined PET/CT to assess regional lymph node involvement in gastric cancer. Tumori 2014;100(2): 201–6.

29. Lee SJ, Lee WW, Yoon HJ, et al. Regional PET/CT after water gastric inflation for evaluating loco-regional disease of gastric cancer. Eur J Radiol 2013;82(6): 935–42.

30. Smyth E, Schoder H, Strong VE, et al. A prospective evaluation of the utility of 2-deoxy-2-[(18) F]fluoro-D-glucose positron emission tomography and computed tomography in staging locally advanced gastric cancer. Cancer 2012;118(22):5481–8.

31. Ma DW, Kim JH, Jeon TJ, et al. (1)(8)F-fluorodeoxyglucose positron emission tomography-computed tomography for the evaluation of bone metastasis

in patients with gastric cancer. Dig Liver Dis 2013; 45(9):769–75.

32. Choi BW, Kim HW, Won KS, et al. Diagnostic accuracy of 18F-FDG PET/CT for detecting synchronous advanced colorectal neoplasia in patients with gastric cancer. Medicine (Baltimore) 2016; 95(36):e4741.

33. Couper GW, McAteer D, Wallis F, et al. Detection of response to chemotherapy using positron emission tomography in patients with oesophageal and gastric cancer. Br J Surg 1998;85(10):1403–6.

34. Kim SJ, Cho YS, Moon SH, et al. Primary tumor (1)(8) F-FDG avidity affects the performance of (1)(8)F-FDG PET/CT for detecting gastric cancer recurrence. J Nucl Med 2016;57(4):544–50.

35. Zou H, Zhao Y. 18FDG PET-CT for detecting gastric cancer recurrence after surgical resection: a meta-analysis. Surg Oncol 2013;22(3):162–6.

36. Wu LM, Hu JN, Hua J, et al. 18 F-fluorodeoxyglucose positron emission tomography to evaluate recurrent gastric cancer: a systematic review and meta-analysis. J Gastroenterol Hepatol 2012;27(3): 472–80.

37. Kim DW, Park SA, Kim CG. Detecting the recurrence of gastric cancer after curative resection: comparison of FDG PET/CT and contrast-enhanced abdominal CT. J Korean Med Sci 2011;26(7):875–80.

38. Nakamoto Y, Togashi K, Kaneta T, et al. Clinical value of whole-body FDG-PET for recurrent gastric cancer: a multicenter study. Jpn J Clin Oncol 2009;39(5):297–302.

39. Sim SH, Kim YJ, Oh DY, et al. The role of PET/CT in detection of gastric cancer recurrence. BMC Cancer 2009;9:73.

40. Lee JW, Lee SM, Lee MS, et al. Role of (1)(8)F-FDG PET/CT in the prediction of gastric cancer recurrence after curative surgical resection. Eur J Nucl Med Mol Imaging 2012;39(9):1425–34.

41. Sharma P, Singh H, Suman SK, et al. 18F-FDG PET-CT for detecting recurrent gastric adenocarcinoma: results from a non-Oriental Asian population. Nucl Med Commun 2012;33(9):960–6.

42. Lee DY, Lee CH, Seo MJ, et al. Performance of (18)F-FDG PET/CT as a postoperative surveillance imaging modality for asymptomatic advanced gastric cancer patients. Ann Nucl Med 2014; 28(8):789–95.

43. Choi BW, Zeon SK, Kim SH, et al. Significance of SUV on Follow-up F-18 FDG PET at the anastomotic site of gastroduodenostomy after distal subtotal gastrectomy in patients with gastric cancer. Nucl Med Mol Imaging 2011;45(4):285–90.

44. Lee JW, Lee SM, Son MW, et al. Diagnostic performance of FDG PET/CT for surveillance in asymptomatic gastric cancer patients after curative surgical resection. Eur J Nucl Med Mol Imaging 2016;43(5): 881–8.

45. Chung HW, Lee EJ, Cho YH, et al. High FDG uptake in PET/CT predicts worse prognosis in patients with metastatic gastric adenocarcinoma. J Cancer Res Clin Oncol 2010;136(12):1929–35.

46. Kim J, Lim ST, Na CJ, et al. Pretreatment F-18 FDG PET/CT parameters to evaluate progression-free survival in gastric cancer. Nucl Med Mol Imaging 2014;48(1):33–40.

47. Park JC, Lee JH, Cheoi K, et al. Predictive value of pretreatment metabolic activity measured by fluoro-deoxyglucose positron emission tomography in patients with metastatic advanced gastric cancer: the maximal SUV of the stomach is a prognostic factor. Eur J Nucl Med Mol Imaging 2012;39(7):1107–16.

48. Park JW, Cho CH, Jeong DS, et al. Role of F-fluoro-2-deoxyglucose positron emission tomography in gastric GIST: predicting malignant potential preoperatively. J Gastric Cancer 2011;11(3):173–9.

49. Grabinska K, Pelak M, Wydmanski J, et al. Prognostic value and clinical correlations of 18-fluorodeoxyglucose metabolism quantifiers in gastric cancer. World J Gastroenterol 2015;21(19):5901–9.

50. Na SJ, O JH, Park JM, et al. Prognostic value of metabolic parameters on preoperative 18F-Fluorodeoxyglucose positron emission tomography/computed tomography in patients with stage III gastric cancer. Oncotarget 2016;7(39):63968–80.

51. Song BI, Kim HW, Won KS, et al. Preoperative standardized uptake value of metastatic lymph nodes measured by 18F-FDG PET/CT improves the prediction of prognosis in gastric cancer. Medicine (Baltimore) 2015;94(26):e1037.

52. Yang QM, Kawamura T, Itoh H, et al. Is PET-CT suitable for predicting lymph node status for gastric cancer? Hepatogastroenterology 2008;55(82–83):782–5.

53. Kim MS, Saunders AM, Hamaoka BY, et al. Structure of the protein core of the glypican Dally-like and localization of a region important for hedgehog signaling. Proc Natl Acad Sci U S A 2011;108(32):13112–7.

54. Filik M, Kir KM, Aksel B, et al. The role of 18F-FDG PET/CT in the primary staging of gastric cancer. Mol Imaging Radionucl Ther 2015;24(1):15–20.

55. Park MJ, Lee WJ, Lim HK, et al. Detecting recurrence of gastric cancer: the value of FDG PET/CT. Abdom Imaging 2009;34(4):441–7.

56. Lee JE, Hong SP, Ahn DH, et al. The role of 18F-FDG PET/CT in the evaluation of gastric cancer recurrence after curative gastrectomy. Yonsei Med J 2011;52(1):81–8.

57. Cayvarli H, Bekis R, Akman T, et al. The role of 18F-FDG PET/CT in the evaluation of gastric cancer recurrence. Mol Imaging Radionucl Ther 2014;23(3):76–83.

58. Li P, Liu Q, Wang C, et al. Fluorine-18-fluorodeoxyglucose positron emission tomography to evaluate recurrent gastric cancer after surgical resection: a systematic review and meta-analysis. Ann Nucl Med 2016;30(3):179–87.

Precision Medicine and PET/Computed Tomography in Melanoma

Esther Mena, MD[a],*, Yasemin Sanli, MD[b],
Charles Marcus, MD[c],
Rathan M. Subramaniam, MD, PhD, MPH[b,d,e,f]

KEYWORDS

- Melanoma • Molecular imaging • Targeted therapy • Immunotherapy • Biomarker
- Precision oncology

KEY POINTS

- Understanding the molecular and genetic alterations in the pathogenesis of melanoma will elucidate the mechanisms involved in tumor growth and aid in the development of potential targeted drugs.
- Future research directions will involve incorporation of molecular characteristics and next-generation probes into new strategies to improve early tumor detection.
- Novel targeted therapies modulating immune inhibitory pathways have revolutionized melanoma, bringing a new exciting approach in the response assessment of melanoma.
- In the context of new targeted therapy, the next steps involve strategies for using PET imaging as a prognostic biomarker to identify patients who could benefit from targeted therapy, predict early identification of responders/nonresponders, and monitor secondary resistances, ultimately leading to improved clinical management, individualizing therapy decisions, and eventually predicting patient outcomes.

INTRODUCTION

Melanoma of the skin represents the sixth most common cancer in the United States, and its incidence has continued to increase over the past few decades.[1] Although many patients with early stage melanoma have favorable outcomes following complete surgical resection, treatment continues to be challenging for patients with advanced metastatic disease.[2] Furthermore, accurate restaging and follow-up therapy assessment becomes crucial for the appropriate management of patients with melanoma, because about 50% to 80% of patients with melanoma with locoregional disease and nearly all patients with distant metastases will experience tumor recurrence after treatment.[3]

Recent interest in understanding the biology and pathogenesis of melanoma has led to the discovery of vital signaling pathways and the

[a] Molecular Imaging Program, National Cancer Institute, National Institutes of Health, 9000 Rockville Pike, Building 10, Room B3B402, Bethesda, MD 20892-1763, USA; [b] Department of Radiology, The University of Texas Southwestern Medical Center, Dallas, TX, USA; [c] The Russell H. Morgan Department of Radiology and Radiological Sciences, The Johns Hopkins University School of Medicine, 601 North Caroline Street, Baltimore, MD 21231, USA; [d] Department of Clinical Sciences, The University of Texas Southwestern Medical Center, 5323 Harry Hines Boulevard, Dallas, TX 75390-8896, USA; [e] Department of Biomedical Engineering, The University of Texas Southwestern Medical Center, 5323 Harry Hines Boulevard, Dallas, TX 75390-8896, USA; [f] Advanced Imaging Research Center, The University of Texas Southwestern Medical Center, 5323 Harry Hines Boulevard, Dallas, TX 75390-8896, USA
* Corresponding author.
E-mail address: esther.menagonzalez@nih.gov

PET Clin 12 (2017) 449–458
http://dx.doi.org/10.1016/j.cpet.2017.05.002
1556-8598/17/Published by Elsevier Inc.

development of mutation-driven therapy, immunotherapy, and targeted therapies, which have revolutionized the clinical history of this disease by dramatically improving the outcomes of patients with metastatic disease. Immunotherapy is mostly based on immune checkpoint inhibitors targeting cytotoxic T-lymphocyte antigen 4 (CTLA-4), and more recently programmed cell death protein 1 (PD-1)/programmed death ligand 1 (PD-L1) interaction.[4] Targeted therapies with mitogen-activated protein kinase (MAPK) pathway kinase inhibitors have also been developed due to the discovery that v-raf murine sarcoma viral oncogene homolog B1 (BRAF) and NRAS mutations, which are among the major oncogenic drivers of melanoma proliferation and survival.[5] As new therapies become available, there is a need to identify biomarkers to guide patient selection, and monitor treatment response. The use of molecular imaging using PET offers unique insights in oncology, helping early tumor detection, characterization, real time monitoring of treatment response, and identification of tumor recurrence. This review summarizes the recent genomic and therapeutic discoveries in melanoma and their implications for imaging.

MOLECULAR GENETICS AND IMMUNOMODULATION IN MELANOMA

The concept of targeting genomic alterations has experienced significant success in oncology, especially in patients with melanoma. Oncogenic targets are genes that are mutated and/or expressed in tumor tissue, contributing to tumor growth and dissemination, and have the potential to be pharmacologically targetable.[6] Investigators at The Cancer Genome Atlas[7] Research Network identified molecular subtypes of melanoma that could potentially guide clinicians to identify the more aggressive tumors and the ones more likely to respond to certain therapies. More than 90% of melanoma tumors harbor activating mutations in oncogenes within the MAPK pathway, which plays a major role in coordinating the balance between melanocyte differentiation and proliferation.[8] Approximately 50% of patients with melanoma are displaying mutations in the harbor BRAF-V600 mutations,[4] about 20% in the NRAS, up to 14% in the NF1 gene, and 3% to 5% harbor an activating KIT mutation.[9,10] These findings have led to the development of BRAF and MEK inhibitors whose applications in the clinic have shown unprecedented survival responses. BRAF blockade therapy with the Food and Drug Administration (FDA)–approved vemurafenib or dabrafenib and also in combination of MEK inhibitor, trametinib, have successfully lead

to an improved progression-free survival (PFS) and overall survival (OS) in patients with the typical BRAF-V600–mutant compared with conventional chemotherapy.[11–13] However, even when treated with the combination, most patients develop mechanisms of drug resistance, without achieving a complete tumor regression. Furthermore, the remaining subset of 50% to 60% of patients with advanced melanoma without a BRAF-V600 mutation, also called BRAF wild-type (BRAF WT), do not benefit from treatment with BRAF inhibitors.

Along with the development of BRAF and MEK inhibitors, immunotherapy has made an important step forward and specifically the immune checkpoint inhibitors. Immunomodulatory strategies use monoclonal antibodies to target key regulators of T-lymphocyte activation and thereby inhibit immune tolerance toward tumor cells.[14] Ipilimumab, a fully human monoclonal antibody that targets anti–CTLA-4, was approved by the FDA in 2011 for first- and second-line treatment of patients with unresectable or advanced melanoma,[15] resulting in significant OS benefit[16] (**Figs. 1–3**). The successes of ipilimumab were quickly followed by trials targeting the immune inhibitor interaction between PD-1, found on T cells, and its ligand (PD-L1) found on tumor cells (**Fig. 4**); pembrolizumab and nivolumab were the first anti–PD-1 pathway family of checkpoint inhibitors to gain accelerated approval from the FDA for the treatment of ipilimumab-refractory melanoma (**Fig. 5**), which demonstrated objective antitumor response rates in up to 45% of treatment-naïve patients with advanced melanoma, with durable long-term survival.[17,18] Furthermore, combined checkpoint blockade with nivolumab plus ipilimumab has demonstrated even greater objective response rates and survival than anti–PD-1 and anti–CTLA-4 monotherapy alone strategies, albeit with significantly more adverse events.[19–21]

All these novel treatment strategies showed promising results for patients with advanced metastatic melanoma; however, they also hold significant challenges because there is no a robust biomarker to identify what subpopulation of patients with melanoma will most likely benefit from one type of treatment or another. Without a predictive biomarker, many patients may receive treatment without benefit. Besides, monitoring the effects of these treatments may also be a challenge because when the immune system is stimulated, immune cells infiltrate the tumor that leads to the cytotoxic effects of the therapy; these immune infiltrates may cause imaging misinterpretations in the response assessment. The following sections outline the

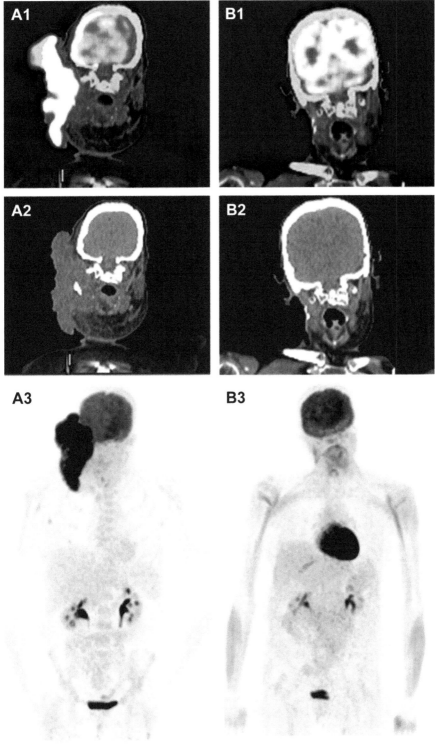

Baseline PET MIP　　**Post-therapy PET MIP**

Fig. 1. Complete metabolic tumor response after combined radiation and ipilimumab treatment in a patient with locally advanced metastatic melanoma: 72-year-old woman diagnosed with locally advanced metastatic malignant melanoma, who underwent combined therapy with radiation plus an immune checkpoint inhibitor, ipilimumab. Baseline fused coronal PET/computed tomography (CT) (*A1*), CT (*A2*), and maximum intensity projection (MIP) (*A3*) images demonstrate a large, intense fluorodeoxyglucose-avid right neck mass. After radiotherapy and 4 cycles of ipilimumab, the fused coronal PET/CT (*B1*), CT (*B2*), and MIP PET (*B3*) images show complete metabolic response.

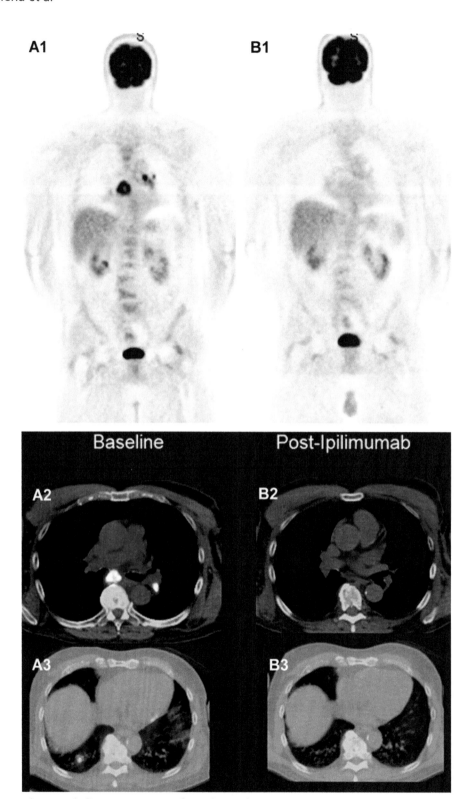

Fig. 2. Complete metabolic tumor response after ipilimumab treatment in a patient with stage IV metastatic melanoma: 68-year-old woman diagnosed with stage IV melanoma. Baseline PET maximum intensity projection (MIP) image (*A1*) and axial fused PET/computed tomography (CT) images (*A2, A3*) demonstrate multiple fluorodeoxyglucose-avid mediastinal nodal lesions (*A2*) and a metastatic pulmonary nodule in the right lung base (*A3*). After 4 cycles of ipilimumab, MIP PET image (*B1*) and axial fused PET/CT images (*B2, B3*) show complete metabolic response.

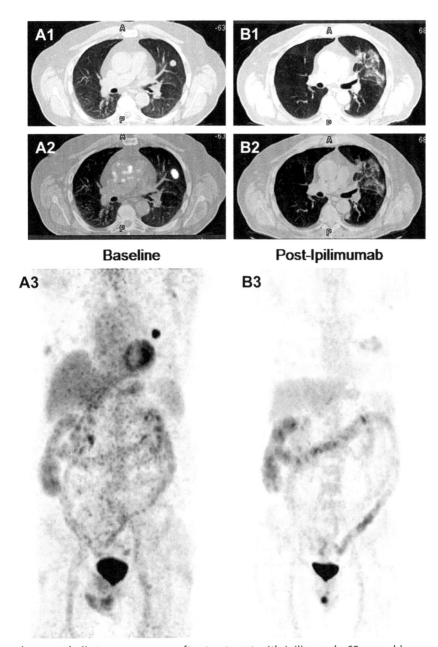

Baseline   **Post-Ipilimumab**

Fig. 3. Complete metabolic tumor response after treatment with ipilimumab: 65-year-old man with stage IV metastatic melanoma. Baseline axial computed tomography (CT) (*A1*), fused PET/CT (*A2*), and maximum intensity projection (MIP) (*A3*) images demonstrate an intense fluorodeoxyglucose (FDG)-avid left upper lobe pulmonary metastatic lesion. After stereotactic body radiation therapy, and concurrent treatment with ipilimumab, the axial CT (*B1*), fused PET/CT (*B2*), and MIP (*B3*) images demonstrate complete metabolic resolution of the lung nodule, with mild FDG-avid radiotherapy inflammatory-related lung changes.

current ways in which PET imaging can be used as a biomarker in patients with melanoma undergoing immune or targeted therapies and how to adapt the imaging interpretation to respond to the unique challenges of immunotherapy.

PET IMAGING IN ASSESSING RESPONSE TO THERAPY IN THE ERA OF PERSONALIZED TREATMENT

As the treatment of cancer evolves to include new agents, attention has been given to how a specific treatment might impact imaging findings.

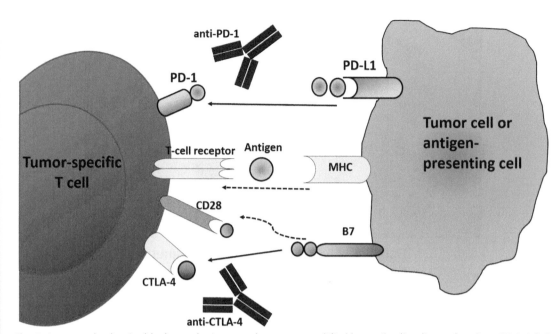

Fig. 4. Immune checkpoint blockage: the immunotherapy exemplified by antibodies directed against CTLA-4 (ipi-limumab, tremelimumab), which block the immunosuppression mediated by the interaction between CTLA-4 (located on the CD8+ and CD4+ T cells) and the B7 family members (located on the antigen-presenting cells). The other second major checkpoint is mediated by the interaction between PD-1 (located on T cells) and its ligand PD-L1 (located on either antigen-presenting cells or on the tumor cells). MHC, major histocompatibility complex.

Fluorine-18 fluorodeoxyglucose (18F-FDG) positron PET/computed tomography (CT) is a powerful imaging tool widely used to evaluate treatment response in multiple malignancies, including melanoma. In the setting of assessing response to mutation-drive therapy, BRAF kinase mutation has been shown to affect multiple signaling pathways, which upregulate glycolysis and glucose transport, facilitating tumor growth.[22,23] Thus, the resultant change in glucose metabolism from targeting mutated BRAF kinase agents could theoretically be visualized using FDG PET/CT. In this context, in a phase I study, including 27 patients with stage IV BRAF-V600 mutation, McArthur and colleagues[24] were able to show, homogeneously, dose-dependent decreased 18F-FDG uptake in metastases 15 days after starting treatment with vemurafenib, confirming the utility of FDG PET imaging in documenting treatment response early on in the course of therapy. The investigators demonstrated that a median reduction in maximum standardized uptake value (SUVmax) of 82% resulted in significantly different median times of PFS; however, no definitive relationship was found between reduction in target lesion SUVmax and best response according to Response Evaluation Criteria in Solid Tumors (RECIST).[24] Similarly, Carlino and colleagues[25] reported that FDG PET/CT registered responses in all 26

patients with BRAF-mutated metastatic melanoma treated with dabrafenib and that 26% of cases exhibited homogeneous PET responses, whereas 74% showed heterogeneous PET responses; defining a homogeneous response as greater than 90% of lesions responded with no progressive metabolic lesions and up to 10% stable lesions allowed, whereas a heterogeneous response was defined when lesions responded alongside with progressing or new lesions.[25] Although these early data are promising, additional studies are required to characterize the PET response characteristics of the mutation-drive melanoma therapies.

To assess if patients are responding to treatment, the RECIST guideline is currently widely used to evaluate antitumor activity of traditional cytotoxic agents. It helps clinicians to objectively determine whether the tumors have progressed (>20% increase in target lesion size), have responded (>30% decrease in target tumor size), or remained stable (based on a set of radiological measurement criteria). However, in the setting of assessing response to immunomodulation, antitumor responses to immunotherapies are unique in that lesions may progress before a documented response,[26] response can be seen in spite of the presence of new lesions, and lesions may remain stable or slowly regress over time, which

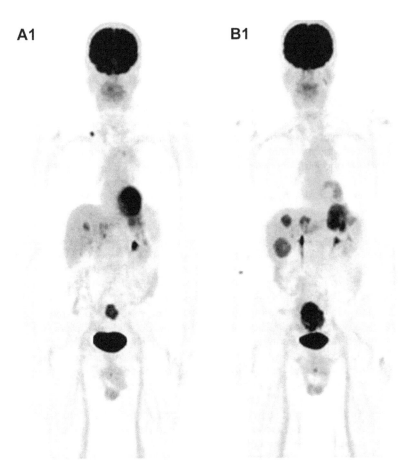

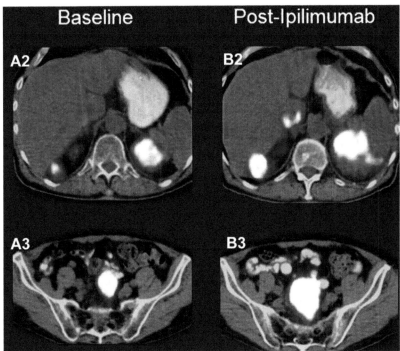

Fig. 5. Ipilimumab-refractory melanoma in a patient with stage IV disease: 72-year-old gentleman diagnosed with stage IV melanoma. Baseline PET maximum intensity projection (MIP) image (*A1*) and axial fused PET/computed tomography images (*A2, A3*) demonstrate multiple fluorodeoxyglucose (FDG)-avid metastatic lesions. After 4 cycles of ipilimumab, MIP PET image (*B1*) shows increase in size and FDG avidity of the prior lesions and development of new FDG-avid lesions (*B2, B3*) indicating progression of metabolic disease.

may take longer than cytotoxic therapies. Immune modulation therapy response can also be confounded by the presence of inflammatory cells, which can mimic FDG-avid tumor,[27] further complicating assessments of therapy response. Another consideration to have in mind when performing FDG PET/CT imaging following immunotherapy is that it potentiates T lymphocytes, producing a high rate (up to 70%) of immune-related adverse reactions, including colitis, dermatitis, hypophysitis, arthritis, and thyroiditis, which can also lead to false findings on FDG PET imaging.[28–35] These effects raise concerns about the use of existing response interpretation criteria, including World Health Organization, RECIST, or PERCIST (Positron Emission Response Criteria In Solid Tumors) criteria[26]; there is a necessity for defining new standard response criteria to assess response to these novel immunotherapies. In a series of workshops in 2004 and 2005, the immune-related response criteria (irRC) was introduced. The irRC incorporates measurable new lesions into a new concept of "total tumor burden" and compares this novel metric with the baseline measurements.[26] Using IrRC criteria, Kong and collaborators[36] recently aimed to described the patterns of residual metabolic activity in patients following prolonged treatment with anti–CTLA-4 or anti–PD-1 antibodies in 27 patients with unresectable stage IIIC or IV melanoma. The data suggested that patients with residual metastases may have metabolically inactive lesions on FDG PET imaging, whereas isolated metabolically active lesions in clinically well patients may reveal immune cell infiltrates rather than melanoma.[36] Moreover, Sachpekidis and colleagues[37] showed that FDG PET/CT imaging may have a role in the early detection of ipilimumab immune-related response in 22 patients with unresectable metastatic melanoma; FDG PET/CT after 2 cycles of ipilimumab was highly predictive of the final treatment outcome in patients with progression and stable metabolic disease.[37] Further prospective studies and long-term follow-up are in need to clarify whether or not FDG PET may be useful as a biomarker of duration of treatment response, early response assessment, and to what extent immune activation can lead to false-positive results.

PET AS A PREDICTIVE BIOMARKER OF PROGNOSIS IN THE NEW-GENERATION THERAPIES

MAPK inhibitors and immunologic checkpoint blockade antibodies have achieved improved OS in patients with metastatic melanoma.[38] There is also evidence that FDG PET/CT findings can be used to prognosticate clinical outcomes after the new-generation mutation-driven therapy and immunomodulation therapy. In the aforementioned phase I study, including 27 patients with BRAF-V600–mutated metastatic melanoma treated with vemurafenib, McArthur and colleagues[24] reported that, although PET response was unrelated to OS, subjects who experienced a reduction in the SUV-max of less than 82% had a mean PFS of 183 days, which was substantially shorter than the 484 days of PFS for those with a greater than 82% reduction in SUVmax. Similarly, Carlino and colleagues,[25] in a phase I study using dabrafenib therapy in BRAF-V600–mutated metastatic melanomas, found that patients with heterogeneous FDG PET responses had a significantly shorter PFS than homogeneous FDG PET responders (mean, 3.0 vs 7.4 months, respectively). In the context of combined BRAF and MEK inhibitor therapy, Schmitt and colleagues[39] investigated the association between survival and early changes on FDG PET/CT imaging in 22 patients with BRAF-mutant melanoma. Investigators found that, for the least metabolically active tumor, change in SUVmax was associated with PFS but not OS; for the least metabolically active tumor, no association was seen between changes in SUVmax and PFS or OS.[39]

In the setting of immunomodulation therapy agents, there are no published data assessing the prognostic benefits of using FDG PET, other than case reports illustrating radiologic features of the immune-related adverse reactions, highlighting the challenges of monitoring immunomodulation therapy with FDG PET. Thus, Bronstein and colleagues[33] reviewed case reports of 119 patients with stage IV melanoma treated with anti–CTLA-4, concluding that there was a significant association between the incidence of radiologic manifestations of immune-related adverse events and clinical responses to anti–CTLA-4 therapy; interestingly, 25% of patients with radiologic manifestation due to immune-related adverse events experienced complete response compared with 3% of patients who did not exhibit radiologic evidence of immune-related adverse events.[33]

FDG PET/CT has also been recently proposed as a potential marker to aid predicting patients' prognosis in different tumors, by using the various PET metabolic parameters, such as the SUVmax, metabolic tumor volume (MTV), and total lesion glycolysis (TLG). SUVmax is a semiquantitative measure of tumor FDG uptake, whereas MTV refers to volumetric measurement of tumor cells with high glycolytic activity; TLG is the sum of SUVs within the tumor, calculated as MTV × SUVmean. In the setting of melanoma, Kang and colleagues[40] reported that the SUVmax from FDG

PET/CT can provide important information for predicting recurrence. Using PET volumetric parameters, Son and colleagues[41] retrospectively conducted a review study including 41 patients with a histologic diagnosis of cutaneous melanoma who underwent pretreatment FDG PET/CT scans; SUVmax and TLG were found to be significantly higher in patients with recurrence than in patients without, and SUVmax and TLG were also found to be significantly higher in nonsurvivors than in survivors. Investigators concluded that pretreatment MTV and TLG may be useful in stratifying the likelihood of recurrence and melanoma-specific death and that TLG was found to be the best predictive marker.[41] Further additional studies are necessary for assessing whether pretreatment or posttreatment FDG PET parameters can predict immunomodulation treatment success.

SUMMARY/DISCUSSION

The molecular classification of cancer through next-generation sequencing has transformed drug development toward the molecularly guided era of precision oncology. With the advances and successes of mutation-driven and immuno-modulation therapy, the ultimate goal is to tailor treatment of specific melanoma subtypes and patients. Treatment response criteria should be chosen based on the subtype of tumor and treatment delivered to patients and should evolve in parallel with the advances in novel targeted agents. As a result, it is crucial that radiologists are aware that the major advancements in cancer immunotherapy are challenging the current imaging approach in evaluating treatment response and early recognizing immune-related adverse events for successful patient management. Further prospective studies and long-term follow-up are needed to determine the role of FDG PET/CT imaging as a potential prognostic biomarker to identify patients suitable for targeted therapy, predict early response assessment, duration of treatment response, monitor secondary resistances, and eventually predicting patient outcome.

REFERENCES

1. Siegel RL, Miller KD, Jemal A. Cancer statistics, 2016. CA Cancer J Clin 2016;66(1):7–30.
2. Balch CM, Gershenwald JE, Soong SJ, et al. Final version of 2009 AJCC melanoma staging and classification. J Clin Oncol 2009;27(36):6199–206.
3. Leiter U, Meier F, Schittek B, et al. The natural course of cutaneous melanoma. J Surg Oncol 2004;86(4):172–8.
4. Ascierto PA, Marincola FM. 2015: the year of anti-PD-1/PD-L1s against melanoma and beyond. EBioMedicine 2015;2(2):92–3.
5. Menzies AM, Long GV. Systemic treatment for BRAF-mutant melanoma: where do we go next? Lancet Oncol 2014;15(9):e371–81.
6. Iams WT, Sosman JA, Chandra S. Novel targeted therapies for metastatic melanoma. Cancer J 2017; 23(1):54–8.
7. Cancer Genome Atlas Network. Genomic classification of cutaneous melanoma. Cell 2015;161(7): 1681–96.
8. Inamdar GS, Madhunapantula SV, Robertson GP. Targeting the MAPK pathway in melanoma: why some approaches succeed and other fail. Biochem Pharmacol 2010;80(5):624–37.
9. Hodis E, Watson IR, Kryukov GV, et al. A landscape of driver mutations in melanoma. Cell 2012;150(2): 251–63.
10. Krauthammer M, Kong Y, Ha BH, et al. Exome sequencing identifies recurrent somatic RAC1 mutations in melanoma. Nat Genet 2012;44(9): 1006–14.
11. Chapman PB, Hauschild A, Robert C, et al. Improved survival with vemurafenib in melanoma with BRAF V600E mutation. N Engl J Med 2011; 364(26):2507–16.
12. Hauschild A, Grob JJ, Demidov LV, et al. Dabrafenib in BRAF-mutated metastatic melanoma: a multicentre, open-label, phase 3 randomised controlled trial. Lancet 2012;380(9839):358–65.
13. Flaherty KT, Robert C, Hersey P, et al. Improved survival with MEK inhibition in BRAF-mutated melanoma. N Engl J Med 2012;367(2):107–14.
14. Ott PA, Hodi FS, Robert C. CTLA-4 and PD-1/PD-L1 blockade: new immunotherapeutic modalities with durable clinical benefit in melanoma patients. Clin Cancer Res 2013;19(19):5300–9.
15. Chmielowski B. Ipilimumab: a first-in-class T-cell potentiator for metastatic melanoma. J Skin Cancer 2013;2013:423829.
16. Hodi FS, O'Day SJ, McDermott DF, et al. Improved survival with ipilimumab in patients with metastatic melanoma. N Engl J Med 2010;363(8):711–23.
17. Topalian SL, Sznol M, McDermott DF, et al. Survival, durable tumor remission, and long-term safety in patients with advanced melanoma receiving nivolumab. J Clin Oncol 2014;32(10):1020–30.
18. Ribas A, Hamid O, Daud A, et al. Association of pembrolizumab with tumor response and survival among patients with advanced melanoma. JAMA 2016;315(15):1600–9.
19. Postow MA, Chesney J, Pavlick AC, et al. Nivolumab and ipilimumab versus ipilimumab in untreated melanoma. N Engl J Med 2015;372(21):2006–17.
20. Larkin J, Chiarion-Sileni V, Gonzalez R, et al. Combined nivolumab and ipilimumab or monotherapy

in untreated melanoma. N Engl J Med 2015;373(1): 23–34.

21. Hodi FS, Chesney J, Pavlick AC, et al. Combined nivolumab and ipilimumab versus ipilimumab alone in patients with advanced melanoma: 2-year overall survival outcomes in a multicentre, randomised, controlled, phase 2 trial. Lancet Oncol 2016; 17(11):1558–68.

22. Zheng B, Jeong JH, Asara JM, et al. Oncogenic B-RAF negatively regulates the tumor suppressor LKB1 to promote melanoma cell proliferation. Mol Cell 2009;33(2):237–47.

23. Kao YS, Fong JC. A novel cross-talk between endothelin-1 and cyclic AMP signaling pathways in the regulation of GLUT1 transcription in 3T3-L1 adipocytes. Cell Signal 2011;23(5):901–10.

24. McArthur GA, Puzanov I, Amaravadi R, et al. Marked, homogeneous, and early [18F]fluorodeoxyglucose-positron emission tomography responses to vemurafenib in BRAF-mutant advanced melanoma. J Clin Oncol 2012;30(14):1628–34.

25. Carlino MS, Saunders CA, Haydu LE, et al. (18)F-labelled fluorodeoxyglucose-positron emission tomography (FDG-PET) heterogeneity of response is prognostic in dabrafenib treated BRAF mutant metastatic melanoma. Eur J Cancer 2013;49(2): 395–402.

26. Wolchok JD, Hoos A, O'Day S, et al. Guidelines for the evaluation of immune therapy activity in solid tumors: immune-related response criteria. Clin Cancer Res 2009;15(23):7412–20.

27. Shozushima M, Tsutsumi R, Terasaki K, et al. Augmentation effects of lymphocyte activation by antigen-presenting macrophages on FDG uptake. Ann Nucl Med 2003;17(7):555–60.

28. Kähler KC, Hauschild A. Treatment and side effect management of CTLA-4 antibody therapy in metastatic melanoma. J Dtsch Dermatol Ges 2011;9(4): 277–86.

29. Lammert A, Schneider HJ, Bergmann T, et al. Hypophysitis caused by ipilimumab in cancer patients: hormone replacement or immunosuppressive therapy. Exp Clin Endocrinol Diabetes 2013;121(10): 581–7.

30. Voskens CJ, Goldinger SM, Loquai C, et al. The price of tumor control: an analysis of rare side effects of anti-CTLA-4 therapy in metastatic melanoma from the ipilimumab network. PLoS One 2013;8(1):e53745.

31. Eckert A, Schoeffler A, Dalle S, et al. Anti-CTLA4 monoclonal antibody induced sarcoidosis in a metastatic melanoma patient. Dermatology 2009;218(1): 69–70.

32. Berman D, Parker SM, Siegel J, et al. Blockade of cytotoxic T-lymphocyte antigen-4 by ipilimumab results in dysregulation of gastrointestinal immunity in patients with advanced melanoma. Cancer Immun 2010;10:11.

33. Bronstein Y, Ng CS, Hwu P, et al. Radiologic manifestations of immune-related adverse events in patients with metastatic melanoma undergoing anti-CTLA-4 antibody therapy. AJR Am J Roentgenol 2011;197(6):W992–1000.

34. Koo PJ, Klingensmith WC, Lewis KD, et al. Anti-CTLA4 antibody therapy related complications on FDG PET/CT. Clin Nucl Med 2014;39(1):e93–6.

35. Gilardi L, Colandrea M, Vassallo S, et al. Ipilimumab-induced immunomediated adverse events: possible pitfalls in (18)F-FDG PET/CT interpretation. Clin Nucl Med 2014;39(5):472–4.

36. Kong BY, Menzies AM, Saunders CA, et al. Residual FDG-PET metabolic activity in metastatic melanoma patients with prolonged response to anti-PD-1 therapy. Pigment Cell Melanoma Res 2016;29(5):572–7.

37. Sachpekidis C, Larribere L, Pan L, et al. Predictive value of early 18F-FDG PET/CT studies for treatment response evaluation to ipilimumab in metastatic melanoma: preliminary results of an ongoing study. Eur J Nucl Med Mol Imaging 2015;42(3):386–96.

38. Spagnolo F, Picasso V, Lambertini M, et al. Survival of patients with metastatic melanoma and brain metastases in the era of MAP-kinase inhibitors and immunologic checkpoint blockade antibodies: a systematic review. Cancer Treat Rev 2016;45:38–45.

39. Schmitt RJ, Kreidler SM, Glueck DH, et al. Correlation between early 18F-FDG PET/CT response to BRAF and MEK inhibition and survival in patients with BRAF-mutant metastatic melanoma. Nucl Med Commun 2016;37(2):122–8.

40. Kang S, Ahn BC, Hong CM, et al. Can (18)F-FDG PET/CT predict recurrence in patients with cutaneous malignant melanoma? Nuklearmedizin 2011; 50(3):116–21.

41. Son SH, Kang SM, Jeong SY, et al. Prognostic value of volumetric parameters measured by pretreatment 18F FDG PET/CT in patients with cutaneous malignant melanoma. Clin Nucl Med 2016;41(6):e266–73.

Precision Medicine and PET/Computed Tomography in Cardiovascular Disorders

Elizabeth H. Dibble, MD*, Don C. Yoo, MD

KEYWORDS

- PET/CT • Cardiovascular disease • Myocardial perfusion imaging • Cardiac viability
- Cardiac sarcoidosis • Cardiac amyloidosis • Infection • Vasculitis

KEY POINTS

- PET myocardial perfusion imaging effectively evaluates coronary vasculature.
- PET/computed tomography (CT) can evaluate for hibernating myocardium in patients who are potential candidates for revascularization procedures.
- PET/CT can evaluate the metabolic and anatomic involvement of a variety of inflammatory, infectious, and malignant cardiovascular disorders.
- PET/CT can identify cardiac involvement in sarcoidosis and amyloidosis.
- Novel targeted radiopharmaceutical agents and novel use of established techniques show promise in diagnosing and monitoring cardiovascular diseases.

INTRODUCTION

Despite advances in prevention, diagnosis, treatment, and understanding of cardiovascular disease, it remains the number 1 cause of death for both men and women in the United States.[1] In addition to heart disease and stroke, which are the leading causes of morbidity and mortality related to cardiovascular disease, inflammatory disorders, amyloidosis, infection, and malignancy can also affect the cardiovascular system.

Advances in imaging have allowed improved noninvasive evaluation of cardiovascular disease. Ultrasonography, MR imaging, and nuclear medicine play critical roles in its evaluation. Over the past 2 decades, single-photon emission computed tomography (SPECT) has been the primary nuclear cardiac imaging technology; use of PET was limited by availability and cost. The past decade has seen increased availability of PET/computed tomography (CT) scanners, primarily used in cancer imaging, which can evaluate metabolic and anatomic involvement of a variety of inflammatory, infectious, and malignant cardiovascular disorders. PET/CT is useful in evaluating coronary vasculature, hibernating myocardium, cardiac sarcoidosis, cardiac amyloidosis, cerebrovascular disease, acute aortic syndromes, cardiac and vascular neoplasms, cardiac and vascular infections, and vasculitis. Novel targeted radiopharmaceutical agents and novel use of established techniques

Disclosures: E.H. Dibble has nothing to disclose; D.C. Yoo is a consultant for Endocyte.
Department of Diagnostic Imaging, The Warren Alpert Medical School of Brown University, Rhode Island Hospital, 593 Eddy Street, Providence, RI 02903, USA
* Corresponding author.
E-mail address: edibble@lifespan.org

show promise in diagnosing and monitoring cardiovascular diseases.

NORMAL ANATOMY AND IMAGING TECHNIQUE
Normal Cardiac Anatomy

The normal heart consists of endocardium, myocardium, epicardium, and pericardium. The right atrium receives venous drainage from the body, and the right ventricle pumps that blood to the lungs for oxygenation. Oxygenated blood returns to the left atrium and is pumped through the body by the left ventricle. The vascular supply to the heart comes from the right coronary artery (RCA) and the left main coronary artery (LM); the LM branches into the left anterior descending artery (LAD) and left circumflex artery. The RCA supplies blood to the inferior left ventricle, the LAD supplies blood to the anterior left ventricle and septum, and the left circumflex artery supplies blood to the lateral and posterior left ventricle.

Cardiac Imaging Techniques

Myocardial perfusion imaging is indicated for patients with known or suspected coronary artery disease. The 2 most commonly used radiopharmaceuticals for PET cardiac perfusion imaging are 82-Rb and 13-N-ammonia. 82-Rb does not require an on-site cyclotron, which is a distinct advantage compared with 13-N-ammonia, which requires an on-site cyclotron. PET myocardial perfusion imaging is faster than SPECT myocardial imaging, has superior attenuation correction, and has higher spatial and temporal resolution. Exercise stress is challenging to perform with PET perfusion radiopharmaceuticals primarily because of the short half-lives. 18F-based tracers have longer half-lives and allow for exercise stress; initial studies have shown promise, but 18F tracers are not yet routinely used.[2] Pharmacologic stress can be performed with adenosine, dipyridamole, regadenoson, or dobutamine.

Cardiac viability imaging is indicated to determine the extent of hibernating myocardium in patients who are potential candidates for revascularization procedures. Viability studies can be performed with 18F fluorodeoxyglucose (FDG) and thallium-201 but FDG is preferred because of its higher spatial resolution and accuracy. Patients are administered a glucose load so that glucose receptors are stimulated to take up FDG. If there is viable tissue in an area of perfusion defect on prior SPECT or PET myocardial perfusion study (ie, hibernating myocardium), it takes up FDG in the corresponding area on viability scan.

Normal Vascular Anatomy (Noncoronary)

The left ventricle pumps blood to the body via the aorta, which branches into progressively smaller arteries, eventually perfusing the body at the level of the capillaries then returning to the heart via the venous system. Arteries are composed of 3 layers: the intima (inner), media (middle), and adventitia (outer). Atherosclerosis affects the intimal layer; other cardiovascular diseases can affect other layers.

Vascular Imaging Techniques

The coronary vasculature can be evaluated by PET perfusion imaging as previously described. In addition, FDG-PET/CT can be used to evaluate for infectious, inflammatory, or neoplastic processes involving the vasculature.

IMAGING PROTOCOLS
Myocardial Perfusion

Myocardial perfusion imaging is indicated for patients with known or suspected coronary artery disease. As previously described, the most common radiopharmaceuticals used for myocardial perfusion imaging are 82-Rb and 13-N-ammonia. Patient preparation includes overnight fasting and avoidance of caffeine and caffeine-containing foods for 24 hours and theophylline-containing medications for 48 hours. Rest images are usually acquired first. Rest and stress images can be acquired on different days; for 2-day studies, stress images are usually acquired first. Scout images are acquired to confirm adequate field of view to cover the heart (standard field of view includes the top of the lung apices to the base of heart). A rest dose of radiopharmaceutical (eg, 30–40 mCi Rb-82) should be administered over 20 to 30 seconds (or the lowest radiation dose necessary to acquire a diagnostic-quality image for the individual PET/CT scanner). An emission scan (typically around 5 minutes) should be obtained for a single bed position. Once a 12-lead electrocardiogram (ECG) is in place and intravenous (IV) access established, the pharmacologic stress agent can be administered (eg, dipyridamole 0.56 mg/kg over 4 minutes). Patients should have ECG, blood pressure, and heart rate monitored. At stress target, a second dose of radiopharmaceutical should be injected (eg, 30–40 mCi Rb-82) followed by an emission scan.

Cardiac Viability

Cardiac viability imaging is indicated for patients who are potential candidates for revascularization procedures and in whom there is suspicion of hibernating myocardium. Studies are performed with a glucose load to push FDG into the myocardium. Contraindications include recent ingestion of food, significant exercise within the prior 24 hours, and increased blood glucose level. Nondiabetic patients should fast for 6 hours before the examination. Patients with diabetes controlled with oral medications should avoid breakfast on the morning of the examination and take regularly scheduled medications. Patients with diabetes who are on insulin should continue their usual diets and medications. On arrival, blood glucose level should be checked with a fingertip stick. If less than 150 mg/dL, 50 g of oral glucose should be administered and FDG can be injected. If blood glucose level is 150 to 200 mg/dL, 25 g of oral glucose should be administered and 2 units of regular insulin should be administered via IV; if blood glucose level is greater than 200 mg/dL, regular insulin should be given via IV. Glucose should be checked again 30 to 40 minutes after glucose or insulin administration and, if it is less than 150 mg/dL, FDG can be administered. The FDG dose should be weight based (typically 0.1–0.15 mCi/kg of FDG depending on the individual PET/CT scanner), should be the lowest dose necessary to acquire a diagnostic-quality image, and it should be administered 60 to 75 minutes before imaging. Parameters for CT acquisition vary by scanner, but scans should be performed at low dose for attenuation correction. Gating can also be performed. CT should cover the cardiac region from the top of the lung apices to the base of heart at a single bed position. Camera setup, patient position, acquisitions, processing, and display for interpretation vary by scanner and software; in our institution, once images have been acquired, they must be reconstructed to provide short axis, horizontal long axis, and vertical long axis views.

Cardiac Sarcoidosis

Cardiac sarcoidosis imaging is indicated for patients with suspected cardiac sarcoidosis. Patient preparation includes fasting (except for water) for at least 6 hours, and preferably 12 hours, to downregulate glucose receptors. Preferred diet before fasting is high fat, high protein, low carbohydrate to maximize free fatty acid metabolism. Nondiabetic patients can take all medications; insulin-dependent diabetic patients should take half of their usual dose on the morning of the test; non–insulin-dependent patients should not take oral diabetes medications on the day of the scan. On arrival, blood glucose level should be checked

with a fingertip stick. If less than 70 mg/dL or greater than 200 mg/dL, the physician should be alerted. If glucose level is acceptable and an IV is established, 10 mCi FDG (or the lowest dose necessary to acquire a diagnostic-quality image) should be administered. After 60 minutes, the patient should be scanned from the top of the lung apices to the base of heart for 10 minutes at a single bed position. This field of view also provides information about nodal status in the chest. If a whole-body sarcoid scan is desired, then the patient can be scanned from the skull to the thighs. A recent study examined the feasibility of using somatostatin receptor–based PET/CT in a small number of patients with suspected cardiac sarcoidosis with promising results, although larger studies are warranted.[3]

Cardiac Amyloidosis

Three radiopharmaceuticals have been approved by the United States Food and Drug Administration (FDA) for imaging amyloid plaques: 18F-florbetapir (Eli Lilly); 18F-flutemetamol (GE Healthcare); and 18F-florbetaben (Piramal Pharma).[4] Although these tracers are typically used for imaging amyloid plaques in the brain in the setting of known or suspected Alzheimer disease, these radiopharmaceuticals (along with 18F-NaF PET/CT) have also been used to image cardiac amyloidosis.[5–9] Because these radiopharmaceuticals are not glucose analogs, fasting is not necessary. The lowest dose necessary to acquire a diagnostic-quality image should be administered; optimal timing of PET image acquisition has not yet been established for amyloid agents[7] and may be shorter for 18F-NaF.[9] The patient should be scanned from the top of the lung apices to the base of heart at a single bed position.

Cardiovascular Infection, Inflammation, and Neoplasm

Whole-body and skull-to-thigh FDG-PET are most commonly used to evaluate malignancy but is also useful in evaluating infection and inflammation. As with other PET imaging, patient preparation includes fasting, avoidance of significant exercise within the prior 24 hours, and having normal blood glucose levels (<200 mg/dL; higher than this level prompts consultation with the attending physician). The radiopharmaceutical dose should be weight based and as low as reasonable to achieve diagnostic-quality imaging. At our institution, we use 0.14 mCi/kg. We use low-dose CT for attenuation correction; as mentioned earlier, specific parameters vary by scanner and radiologist preference. At our institution, all patients are scanned at 120 kV, 5 mm × 5 mm helical acquisition, 0.5-second rotation, and dose modulation. Scan length and tube current vary based on patient size. Patients are scanned approximately 75 minutes after radiopharmaceutical injection; at 65 to 70 minutes after injections, patients should empty their bladders. Once positioned on the table, a CT scout and localizer scan is performed, and the PET scan is performed of the corresponding anatomy (skull to thighs [eg, most staging or restaging malignancy scans] versus whole body [eg, melanoma, cutaneous lymphoma, fever of unknown origin]).

Table 1 summarizes PET/CT cardiovascular imaging protocols.

IMAGING FINDINGS/PATHOLOGY
Cardiac/Pericardiac Imaging

Perfusion
Normal myocardial perfusion rest images should show radiopharmaceutical uptake throughout the myocardium. A defect on rest imaging could be caused by a fixed defect from prior myocardial infarction or artifact. Stress images are acquired after patients are injected with radiopharmaceutical at the designated target time (adenosine, dipyridamole, or regadenoson) or target heart rate (dobutamine). Normal stress images without perfusion defects imply no hemodynamically significant narrowing of the coronary arteries. A perfusion defect of the inferior wall implies RCA narrowing; a perfusion defect of the anterior wall, septum, and/or apex implies LAD narrowing; and a perfusion defect of the anterolateral or inferolateral wall implies left circumflex narrowing.

Viability
Areas of hibernating myocardium, or viable tissue, take up FDG on a viability scan in areas of fixed defect seen on prior perfusion imaging. In contrast, areas of scar/infarct (ie, nonviable tissue) do not take up FDG on viability scan in areas of fixed defect on perfusion imaging (**Fig. 1**).

Nonischemic cardiomyopathies and inflammatory disorders
Sarcoidosis Sarcoidosis is characterized by accumulation of noncaseating granulomas caused by an inciting pathogen or environmental agent[10] that can affect multiple organ systems. Cardiac sarcoidosis can manifest as cardiomyopathy or arrhythmias and is difficult to diagnose on biopsy. Twenty-five percent of patients with sarcoidosis have cardiac involvement on autopsy, although approximately 80% is clinically occult.[11] It can involve the pericardium, myocardium, and endocardium of atria or ventricles; the lateral left ventricular wall at the heart base is affected most commonly followed by the basal septum, with a tendency to involve the conducting system; however, myocardial involvement is usually patchy, which likely contributes to the low diagnostic yield on biopsy.[10] Inflammation from granulomas can eventually lead to scarring. PET/CT can detect early myocardial inflammation before myocardial impairment occurs[12]; it can also show involvement of lung parenchyma and mediastinal lymph nodes. Sarcoid imaging evaluates whether defects on resting perfusion scans are caused by infarct or inflammation; areas of defect on rest perfusion imaging with corresponding uptake on sarcoid imaging suggest inflammation caused by myocardial sarcoidosis (**Fig. 2**). PET also shows promise in detecting sarcoidosis treatment response.[13,14]

Nonischemic inflammatory cardiomyopathies PET/CT has shown other nonischemic inflammatory cardiomyopathies, including inflammatory myocarditis[15] and stress myocardial stunning, or Takotsubo cardiomyopathy. The mechanism of Takotsubo cardiomyopathy is unknown but is likely related to increased catecholamine levels and stress-related neuropeptides, which may cause vascular spasm or myocyte injury.[16]

Amyloidosis Amyloidosis is caused by abnormal folding of extracellular proteins that form pathologic deposits of amyloid plaques.[17] As discussed earlier, 3 radiopharmaceuticals have been approved by the FDA for imaging amyloid plaques in the setting of known or suspected Alzheimer disease, but they (along with 18F-NaF PET/CT) have also been used to image cardiac amyloidosis, which can cause restrictive cardiomyopathy and heart failure.[5–9] Targeted agents may be able to differentiate myocardial thickening caused by amyloidosis from that caused by hypertensive heart disease,[7] and 18F-NaF PET may be able to differentiate transthyretin-related cardiac amyloidosis from the light-chain cardiac amyloidosis,[9] which is typically associated with poorer outcomes.[18] Imaging findings are specific cardiac uptake with amyloid agents or uptake over mediastinal background with NaF PET/CT.

Neoplasm
The most common primary cardiac neoplasm is the myxoma, and the most common primary cardiac malignancy is sarcoma; however, secondary cardiac malignancies are approximately 40 times more common than primary cardiac malignancies[15] (**Fig. 3**). FDG-avid primary and metastatic cardiac malignancies show focal FDG uptake in the heart, and the heart must be windowed appropriately to minimize background myocardial

Table 1
Imaging protocols

Imaging Technique	Indications	Patient Preparation	Radiopharmaceutical	Wait Time Before Scan	Scan Protocol
Myocardial perfusion	Suspected coronary artery disease	Overnight fast, avoidance of caffeine and caffeine-containing foods for 24 h and theophylline-containing medications for 48 h	82-Rb 13-N-ammonia	None	Scout, inject, scan, stress, inject, scan
Cardiac viability	Planned revascularization with suspected hibernating myocardium	Short fast, oral glucose administration	18F-FDG	60 min	Inject, scout, scan
Cardiac sarcoidosis	Sarcoidosis with suspected cardiac involvement	Prolonged fast, high fat, high protein, low carb	18F-FDG	60 min	Inject, scout, scan
Cardiac Amyloidosis	Amyloidosis with suspected cardiac involvement	None with amyloid agents, prolonged fast with NaF	18F-florbetapir 18F-flutemetamol 18F-florbetaben 18F-NaF	30–60 min	Inject, scout, scan
Whole-body PET/CT	Malignancy, inflammation including atherosclerosis, infection	Prolonged fast to evaluate suspected cardiac malignancy	18F-FDG	60 min	Inject, scout, scan

Abbreviation: carb, carbohydrate.

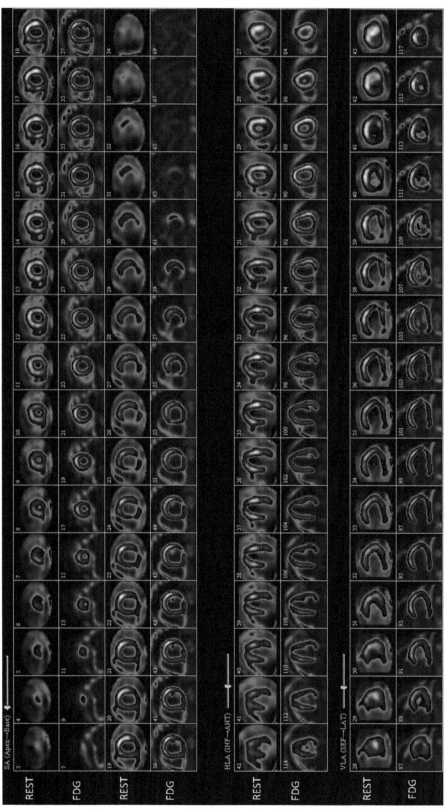

Fig. 1. Rest images from a technetium (Tc)-99m tetrofosmin perfusion study show severe defects in the mid to basal inferior wall. FDG-PET images show predominantly matched defects with only minimal mismatch in the basal inferoseptal wall indicating that most of the defects are nonviable myocardium and the patient will not benefit from revascularization.

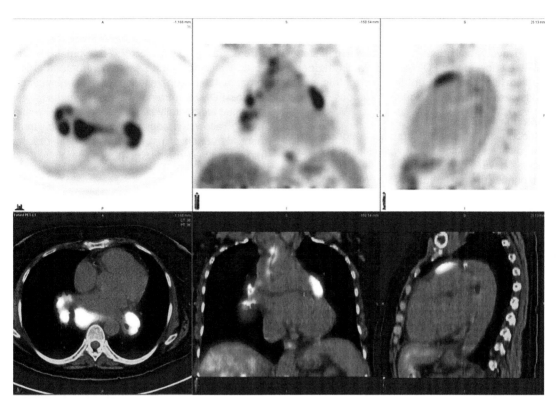

Fig. 2. Axial (*left*), coronal (*middle*), and sagittal (*right*) FDG-PET images in a patient worked up for cardiac sarcoidosis show intense uptake in mediastinal and hilar adenopathy consistent with known sarcoidosis. There is no increased uptake in the left ventricular wall greater than background cardiac blood pool activity to indicate cardiac involvement with sarcoidosis. Rest images from a Tc-99m tetrofosmin perfusion study were normal (not shown).

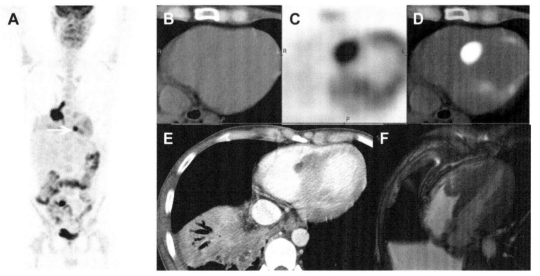

Fig. 3. Maximum intensity projection image (*A*) after IV administration of FDG shows an intensely hypermetabolic focus in the right lung representing the patient's known lung cancer and linear intense uptake in the right hilum/right aspect of the mediastinum. There is a discrete focus of intense activity in the heart (*white arrow*). Axial PET (*C*) and PET/CT (*D*) images centered at the focally increased activity show an intense focus of increased uptake in the interventricular septum without corresponding abnormality on CT (*B*). Contrast-enhanced CT (*E*) shows subtle hypodensity in the interventricular septum. MR imaging (*F*) confirms a mass arising from the interventricular septum. This mass was biopsied and confirmed to represent metastasis.

uptake. Longer fasting and a low-carbohydrate, high-fat, high-protein diet may be helpful in minimizing myocardial uptake.[19] Pericardial metastatic disease shows focal FDG activity within the pericardium. Lack of FDG uptake in an intracardiac mass seen on CT may suggest thrombus.[20]

Infection

Although the ability to diagnose endocarditis in native valves is limited by low sensitivity,[21] recent studies have shown promise in the ability of PET to diagnose prosthetic valve infection and infections of implanted electronic devices.[21–23] PET has also shown endocarditis caused by infected atrial septal defect surgical patch closure.[24] Extracardiac embolic infections can be identified in the setting of endocarditis; one study with 72 patients showed clinically important new findings (not identified by standard work-up) in 1 out of 7 patients imaged with PET/CT.[25] PET has also shown infectious myocarditis, typically in patients with cancer.[15]

Vascular Imaging

Atherosclerosis

Although myocardial perfusion imaging can show altered myocardial metabolism caused by altered coronary blood flow, PET/CT can also directly show atherosclerotic plaque by assessing arterial FDG uptake related to inflammation[26–28] from activated intimal macrophages[29] (symptomatic, unstable plaques show increased uptake compared with asymptomatic plaques[30]) or molecular cardiovascular calcification with 18F NaF PET/CT.[31–33] Inflammation and calcification may represent distinct pathophysiologic processes in the development of atherosclerosis,[34,35] and PET can assess both processes. Protocol alterations to minimize background cardiac uptake may improve visualization of coronary arterial atherosclerotic plaque.[36,37] Recent research has shown the potential of novel PET tracers to target the vascular cell adhesion molecule (VCAM)-1, a molecule implicated in atherosclerosis, by labeling anti–VCAM-1 nanobody (cAbVCAM-1-5) with 18F.[38]

PET may be useful in monitoring response to intervention for atherosclerosis and has shown decreased FDG uptake by atherosclerotic plaques in patients treated with simvastatin compared with diet modification alone.[39]

Aneurysm

Aortic aneurysms can show FDG uptake related to inflammation and macrophage accumulation; FDG uptake may suggest an unstable aneurysm at risk of causing pain, expanding, and/or rupturing versus a stable aneurysm without FDG uptake, which may have a more benign course.[29,40]

Dissection and intramural hematoma

Similarly, there is more uptake in acute versus chronic aortic dissection.[41] FDG uptake in the aortic wall also can be seen in intramural hematoma; platelets adhere to leukocytes, which accumulate FDG.[29] Intramural hematoma has been identified incidentally on PET performed for malignancy, allowing earlier diagnosis and treatment.[29,42] Lack of uptake may suggest that the hematoma is chronic (**Fig. 4**).

Vasculitis

Aortic vasculitis results from accumulation of inflammatory cells in the media (giant cell arteritis and Takayasu arteritis) or periaorta (inflammatory abdominal aortic aneurysms).[29] PET can show active inflammation related to large vessel inflammatory arthritides and may be helpful in monitoring disease activity[43] (**Fig. 5**). Increased vascular activity also can be seen in the setting of systemic inflammatory conditions, including psoriasis and rheumatoid arthritis, even when adjusting for cardiovascular risk factors.[44–46]

Cerebrovascular disease

Using 15-O and 11-C radiopharmaceuticals, PET can image cerebral circulation and metabolism in the setting of stroke and can provide information about ischemic penumbra for intervention planning,[47] although the need for an on-site cyclotron and advances in MR imaging have limited its use. PET is also useful in distinguishing vascular dementia from other neurodegenerative disorders[47] based on the distribution of altered metabolism. Cerebrovascular disease is characterized by decreased uptake with distinct margins in 1 or more vascular territorial distributions or multifocal areas of hypometabolism caused by small infarcts or small vessel disease. PET can also show altered metabolism and/or altered blood flow in the setting of intracerebral hemorrhage.[47]

Infection

PET/CT can identify vascular graft infections; the most suspicious findings are focal and intense FDG uptake, particularly in the setting of fluid collection or abscess formation.[48] PET/CT can also monitor response of graft infections to therapy[49] and complications, for example, fistula to bone causing osteomyelitis.[50] PET/CT has also been used to help diagnose involvement of abdominal aortic aneurysms and aortoiliac reconstructions in patients with *Coxiella burnetii*.[51]

Neoplasm

Although primary vascular tumors are rare, PET/CT has been helpful in the diagnosing and staging

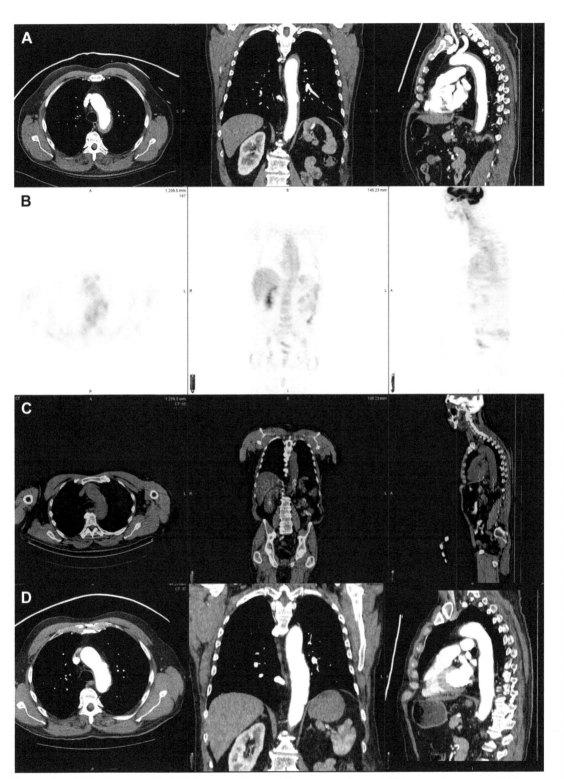

Fig. 4. (*A*) Axial (*left*), coronal (*middle*), and sagittal (*right*) contrast-enhanced CT images show a type B intramural hematoma. PET/CT was performed because there was clinical concern that the patient could have a vasculitis. (*B*, *C*) FDG-PET images show only minimal activity within the aortic wall consistent with intramural hematoma and not a vasculitis. (*D*) Follow-up contrast-enhanced CT images 4 months after the PET/CT scan show resolution of the intramural hematoma.

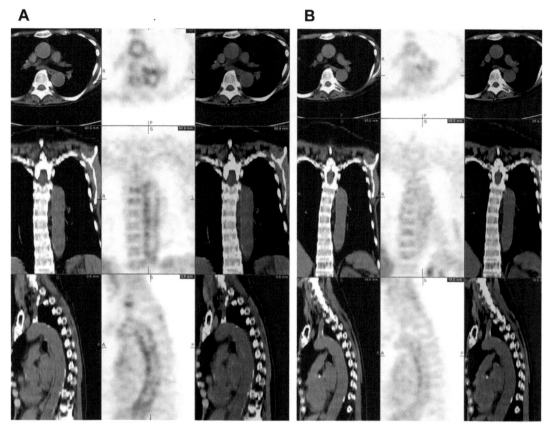

Fig. 5. (*A*) Axial (*top*), coronal (*middle*), and sagittal (*bottom*) CT (*left*), PET (*middle*), and PET/CT (*right*) images of the chest show intense circumferential activity throughout the wall of the thoracic aorta with only minimal atherosclerotic disease seen in the thoracic aorta. (*B*) After treatment with corticosteroids, the circumferential activity in the wall of the thoracic aorta is no longer seen on the PET images.

sarcomas of the great vessels.[52,53] 68Ga-DOTA-NOC (68Ga-labelled [1,4,7,10-tetraazacyclododecane-1,4,7,10-tetraacetic acid]-1-Nal3-octreotide) PET/CT has shown mesenteric vascular thrombosis with a pancreatic neuroendocrine carcinoma.[54]

Diagnostic Criteria

Atherosclerosis

In the setting of suspected atherosclerosis with cardiac risk factors, diagnosis of atherosclerosis on myocardial perfusion imaging requires a perfusion defect in a vascular territory on stress imaging that is not present on rest imaging. Atherosclerosis can also show increased activity in the wall of a blood vessel caused by inflammation or the presence of targeted molecules related to atherosclerosis.

Hibernating myocardium

In the setting of suspected hibernating myocardium in patients who are potential candidates for revascularization procedures, criteria to diagnose hibernating myocardium or viable tissue on imaging include uptake of FDG on viability scan in areas that did not show uptake in comparable SPECT or PET perfusion imaging. Lack of uptake on viability scan suggests myocardial scar or infarct rather than hibernating myocardium.

Cardiac sarcoidosis

In the setting of known or suspected sarcoidosis, myocardial involvement by sarcoidosis can be diagnosed when patchy increased activity is identified, most commonly involving the left ventricle or septum.

Cardiac amyloidosis

Diagnostic criteria include specific cardiac uptake with amyloid agents or uptake over mediastinal background with NaF.

Cerebrovascular disease

Cerebrovascular disease can be diagnosed when PET shows decreased uptake with distinct margins in 1 or more vascular territorial distributions or multifocal areas of decreased uptake, presumably caused by small infarcts/small vessel disease.

Acute aortic syndromes

Increased activity involving an aortic aneurysm, dissection, or intramural hematoma may suggest acuity of findings; lack of uptake suggests a more benign course.

Cardiac or vascular neoplasm

Focal increased activity in the heart, particularly in the setting of known metastatic primary cancer, suggests cardiac metastasis. Focal increased activity associated with a mass in the heart or vasculature without a known malignancy suggests a primary neoplasm.

Cardiac or vascular infection

In the setting of suspected infection (eg, fever, bacteremia), prosthetic valve or implanted electronic device infections show increased activity in the affected area. Vascular graft infection shows focal and intense FDG uptake and is particularly suspicious in the setting of fluid collection or abscess formation.

Vasculitis

Linear or circumferential uptake along blood vessel walls, typically more diffuse than that seen in atherosclerosis, can suggest inflammatory vasculitis and can delineate the extent and distribution of involvement. Findings are particularly suggestive in the setting of a known inflammatory syndrome.

Diagnostic criteria are summarized in **Table 2**.

Differential Diagnosis

Atherosclerosis

On myocardial perfusion imaging, cardiac metastatic lesions can mimic perfusion defects[55] and motion artifact and errors in attenuation correction can mimic defects.

On whole-body PET/CT imaging, uptake caused by vasculitis can mimic atherosclerosis.

Hibernating myocardium

If proper diet preparation is not heeded, hibernating myocardium may be mistaken for myocardial infarction.

Cardiac sarcoidosis

Cardiac tumor can mimic the patchy myocardial involvement of sarcoidosis. Late-stage sarcoidosis may have uptake that is similar or decreased compared with normal myocardium, thus appearing falsely negative on PET imaging.

Cardiac amyloidosis

Targeted amyloid PET imaging agents are specific for identification of amyloid plaques. Further studies are needed to differentiate subtypes of amyloidosis and confirm that imaging findings correlate histologically with plaque burden and ultimately with clinical significance.

Table 2
Diagnostic criteria

Diagnosis	Diagnostic Criteria
Atherosclerosis	Perfusion defect in a vascular territory on stress imaging but not on rest imaging; linear uptake along blood vessel wall
Hibernating myocardium	Radiopharmaceutical uptake in areas without corresponding uptake on perfusion imaging
Cardiac sarcoidosis	Patchy increased myocardial uptake, typically involving the left ventricle or septum
Cardiac amyloidosis	Specific cardiac uptake with amyloid agents or uptake over mediastinal background with NaF
Cerebrovascular disease	Decreased uptake with distinct margins in 1 or more vascular territorial distributions or multifocal areas of hypometabolism caused by small infarcts or small vessel disease
Acute aortic syndromes	Increased uptake involving an aortic aneurysm, dissection, or intramural hematoma may suggest acuity of findings; lack of uptake suggests a more benign course
Cardiac or vascular neoplasm	Focal increased uptake in the heart in the setting of known metastatic disease; focal increased uptake associated with a mass in the heart or vasculature
Cardiac or vascular infection	Focal intense uptake particularly when associated with prosthetic valve, implanted electronic device, or vascular graft in the appropriate clinical setting
Vasculitis	Linear or circumferential uptake along blood vessel walls

Cerebrovascular disease

Multifocal decreased uptake can be seen in the setting of prior insult (eg, hemorrhage, trauma, encephalitis), metastatic disease, or errors in attenuation correction.

Acute aortic syndromes

Uptake in aortic aneurysm, dissection, or intramural hematoma could be caused by infection or vasculitis.

Cardiac or vascular neoplasm

PET/CT uptake with FDG and some other radiopharmaceuticals is nonspecific for infection, inflammation, or malignancy, so abnormal or focal activity must be interpreted in the appropriate clinical setting.

Differential considerations for suspected cardiac neoplasm include normal variation in myocardial activity, uptake in the left atrial appendage, and lipomatous hypertrophy of the intra-atrial septum. Although lipomatous hypertrophy of the intra-atrial septum can show increased FDG activity and enlargement of the intra-atrial septum resembling a neoplastic process, corresponding fat density on CT confirms the diagnosis.

Differential considerations for focal vascular uptake include atherosclerosis, aneurysm, dissection, intramural hematoma, and infection.

Cardiac or vascular infection

As previously described, PET/CT uptake with FDG and some other radiopharmaceuticals is nonspecific for infection, inflammation, or malignancy so must be interpreted in the appropriate clinical setting. Vascular grafts can show uptake related to chronic inflammation and thrombus[29,48] versus infection.

Vasculitis

The differential for vasculitis is atherosclerotic uptake.

Differential diagnoses are summarized in **Table 3**.

Pearls, Pitfalls, Variants

- FDG-PET is nonspecific for infection, inflammation, and malignancy and studies must be interpreted in the appropriate clinical setting
- Motion artifact can mimic lesions; non–attenuation-corrected images may be helpful, particularly in the brain and heart
- Stress must be adequate for myocardial perfusion imaging to avoid false-negatives
- Proper dietary preparation is essential to maximize study yield
- Images should be properly windowed to identify cardiac neoplasms
- Knowledge of normal variants and common benign findings is essential for accurate interpretation; common variants include lipomatous hypertrophy of the intra-atrial septum and vascular graft uptake

What Referring Physicians Need to Know

- PET/CT myocardial perfusion imaging effectively evaluates the coronary vasculature
- Viability PET/CT can evaluate for hibernating myocardium in patients who are potential candidates for revascularization procedures
- PET/CT can evaluate the metabolic and anatomic involvement of a variety of inflammatory, infectious, and malignant cardiovascular disorders
- PET/CT can identify cardiac involvement in sarcoidosis and amyloidosis
- Novel targeted radiopharmaceutical agents and novel use of established techniques show promise in diagnosing and monitoring cardiovascular diseases

Table 3
Differential diagnoses

Diagnosis	Differential Diagnoses
Atherosclerosis	Metastases, vasculitis
Hibernating myocardium	Myocardial infarction
Cardiac sarcoidosis	Tumor
Cardiac amyloidosis	Subtypes of cardiac amyloidosis
Cerebrovascular disease	Prior insult, metastases
Acute aortic syndromes	Infection, vasculitis
Cardiac or vascular neoplasm	Infection, inflammation, atherosclerosis, normal/benign uptake
Cardiac or vascular infection	Inflammation, malignancy

SUMMARY

PET/CT can evaluate the metabolic and anatomic involvement of a variety of inflammatory, infectious, and malignant cardiovascular disorders. PET/CT is useful in evaluating coronary vasculature, hibernating myocardium, cardiac sarcoidosis, cardiac amyloidosis, cerebrovascular disease, acute aortic syndromes, cardiac and vascular neoplasms, cardiac and vascular infections, and vasculitis. Novel targeted radiopharmaceutical agents and novel use of established techniques show promise in diagnosing and monitoring cardiovascular diseases.

REFERENCES

1. Mozaffarian D, Benjamin EJ, Go AS, et al. Heart disease and stroke statistics–2015 update: a report from the American Heart Association. Circulation 2015;131(4):e29–322.
2. Brunken RC. Promising new 18F-labeled tracers for PET myocardial perfusion imaging. J Nucl Med 2015;56(10):1478–9.
3. Lapa C, Reiter T, Kircher M, et al. Somatostatin receptor based PET/CT in patients with the suspicion of cardiac sarcoidosis: an initial comparison to cardiac MRI. Oncotarget 2016;7(47):77807–14.
4. Minoshima S, Drzezga AE, Barthel H, et al. SNMMI procedure standard/EANM practice guideline for amyloid PET imaging of the brain 1.0. J Nucl Med 2016;57(8):1316–22.
5. Lhommel R, Sempoux C, Ivanoiu A, et al. Is 18F-flutemetamol PET/CT able to reveal cardiac amyloidosis? Clin Nucl Med 2014;39(8):747–9.
6. Garcia-Gonzalez P, Cozar-Santiago MD, Maceira AM. Cardiac amyloidosis detected using 18F-florbetapir PET/CT. Rev Esp Cardiol (Engl Ed) 2016;69(12):1215.
7. Law WP, Wang WY, Moore PT, et al. Cardiac amyloid imaging with 18F-florbetaben PET: a pilot study. J Nucl Med 2016;57(11):1733–9.
8. Gagliardi C, Tabacchi E, Bonfiglioli R, et al. Does the etiology of cardiac amyloidosis determine the myocardial uptake of [18F]-NaF PET/CT? J Nucl Cardiol 2017;24(2):746–9.
9. Van Der Gucht A, Galat A, Rosso J, et al. [18F]-NaF PET/CT imaging in cardiac amyloidosis. J Nucl Cardiol 2016;23(4):846–9.
10. Skali H, Schulman AR, Dorbala S. 18F-FDG PET/CT for the assessment of myocardial sarcoidosis. Curr Cardiol Rep 2013;15(4):352.
11. Iannuzzi MC, Rybicki BA, Teirstein AS. Sarcoidosis. N Engl J Med 2007;357(21):2153–65.
12. Okumura W, Iwasaki T, Toyama T, et al. Usefulness of fasting 18F-FDG PET in identification of cardiac sarcoidosis. J Nucl Med 2004;45(12):1989–98.
13. Ahmadian A, Pawar S, Govender P, et al. The response of FDG uptake to immunosuppressive treatment on FDG PET/CT imaging for cardiac sarcoidosis. J Nucl Cardiol 2017;24(2):413–24.
14. Miller CT, Sweiss NJ, Lu Y. FDG PET/CT evidence of effective treatment of cardiac sarcoidosis with adalimumab. Clin Nucl Med 2016;41(5):417–8.
15. Maurer AH, Burshteyn M, Adler LP, et al. How to differentiate benign versus malignant cardiac and paracardiac 18F FDG uptake at oncologic PET/CT. Radiographics 2011;31(5):1287–305.
16. Wittstein IS, Thiemann DR, Lima JA, et al. Neurohumoral features of myocardial stunning due to sudden emotional stress. N Engl J Med 2005;352(6):539–48.
17. Merlini G, Bellotti V. Molecular mechanisms of amyloidosis. N Engl J Med 2003;349(6):583–96.
18. Sperry BW, Vranian MN, Hachamovitch R, et al. Subtype-specific interactions and prognosis in cardiac amyloidosis. J Am Heart Assoc 2016;5(3):e002877.
19. Williams G, Kolodny GM. Suppression of myocardial 18F-FDG uptake by preparing patients with a high-fat, low-carbohydrate diet. AJR Am J Roentgenol 2008;190(2):W151–6.
20. Rinuncini M, Zuin M, Scaranello F, et al. Differentiation of cardiac thrombus from cardiac tumor combining cardiac MRI and 18F-FDG-PET/CT imaging. Int J Cardiol 2016;212:94–6.
21. Yan J, Zhang C, Niu Y, et al. The role of 18F-FDG PET/CT in infectious endocarditis: a systematic review and meta-analysis. Int J Clin Pharmacol Ther 2016;54(5):337–42.
22. Pizzi MN, Roque A, Fernandez-Hidalgo N, et al. Improving the diagnosis of infective endocarditis in prosthetic valves and intracardiac devices with 18F-fluordeoxyglucose positron emission tomography/computed tomography angiography: initial results at an infective endocarditis referral center. Circulation 2015;132(12):1113–26.
23. Granados U, Fuster D, Pericas JM, et al. Diagnostic accuracy of 18F-FDG PET/CT in infective endocarditis and implantable cardiac electronic device infection: a cross-sectional study. J Nucl Med 2016;57(11):1726–32.
24. Honnorat E, Seng P, Riberi A, et al. Late infectious endocarditis of surgical patch closure of atrial septal defects diagnosed by 18F-fluorodeoxyglucose gated cardiac computed tomography (18F-FDG-PET/CT): a case report. BMC Res Notes 2016;9(1):416.
25. Asmar A, Ozcan C, Diederichsen AC, et al. Clinical impact of 18F-FDG-PET/CT in the extra cardiac work-up of patients with infective endocarditis. Eur Heart J Cardiovasc Imaging 2014;15(9):1013–9.
26. Ben-Haim S, Kupzov E, Tamir A, et al. Changing patterns of abnormal vascular wall F-18 fluorodeoxyglucose uptake on follow-up PET/CT studies. J Nucl Cardiol 2006;13(6):791–800.

27. Mehta NN, Torigian DA, Gelfand JM, et al. Quantification of atherosclerotic plaque activity and vascular inflammation using [18-F] fluorodeoxyglucose positron emission tomography/computed tomography (FDG-PET/CT). J Vis Exp 2012;(63): e3777.

28. Pasha AK, Moghbel M, Saboury B, et al. Effects of age and cardiovascular risk factors on (18)F-FDG PET/CT quantification of atherosclerosis in the aorta and peripheral arteries. Hell J Nucl Med 2015;18(1):5–10.

29. Hayashida T, Sueyoshi E, Sakamoto I, et al. PET features of aortic diseases. AJR Am J Roentgenol 2010; 195(1):229–33.

30. Rudd JH, Warburton EA, Fryer TD, et al. Imaging atherosclerotic plaque inflammation with [18F]-fluorodeoxyglucose positron emission tomography. Circulation 2002;105(23):2708–11.

31. Basu S, Beheshti M, Alavi A. Value of (18)F NaF PET/CT in the detection and global quantification of cardiovascular molecular calcification as part of the atherosclerotic process. PET Clin 2012;7(3):329–39.

32. Basu S, Hoilund-Carlsen PF, Alavi A. Assessing global cardiovascular molecular calcification with 18F-fluoride PET/CT: will this become a clinical reality and a challenge to CT calcification scoring? Eur J Nucl Med Mol Imaging 2012;39(4):660–4.

33. Janssen T, Bannas P, Herrmann J, et al. Association of linear (1)(8)F-sodium fluoride accumulation in femoral arteries as a measure of diffuse calcification with cardiovascular risk factors: a PET/CT study. J Nucl Cardiol 2013;20(4):569–77.

34. Derlin T, Toth Z, Papp L, et al. Correlation of inflammation assessed by 18F-FDG PET, active mineral deposition assessed by 18F-fluoride PET, and vascular calcification in atherosclerotic plaque: a dual-tracer PET/CT study. J Nucl Med 2011;52(7): 1020–7.

35. Dunphy MP, Freiman A, Larson SM, et al. Association of vascular 18F-FDG uptake with vascular calcification. J Nucl Med 2005;46(8):1278–84.

36. Wykrzykowska J, Lehman S, Williams G, et al. Imaging of inflamed and vulnerable plaque in coronary arteries with 18F-FDG PET/CT in patients with suppression of myocardial uptake using a low-carbohydrate, high-fat preparation. J Nucl Med 2009;50(4):563–8.

37. Harisankar CN, Mittal BR, Agrawal KL, et al. Utility of high fat and low carbohydrate diet in suppressing myocardial FDG uptake. J Nucl Cardiol 2011;18(5): 926–36.

38. Bala G, Blykers A, Xavier C, et al. Targeting of vascular cell adhesion molecule-1 by 18F-labelled nanobodies for PET/CT imaging of inflamed atherosclerotic plaques. Eur Heart J Cardiovasc Imaging 2016;17(9):1001–8.

39. Tahara N, Kai H, Ishibashi M, et al. Simvastatin attenuates plaque inflammation: evaluation by fluorodeoxyglucose positron emission tomography. J Am Coll Cardiol 2006;48(9):1825–31.

40. Sakalihasan N, Hustinx R, Limet R. Contribution of PET scanning to the evaluation of abdominal aortic aneurysm. Semin Vasc Surg 2004;17(2): 144–53.

41. Reeps C, Pelisek J, Bundschuh RA, et al. Imaging of acute and chronic aortic dissection by 18F-FDG PET/CT. J Nucl Med 2010;51(5):686–91.

42. Ryan A, McCook B, Sholosh B, et al. Acute intramural hematoma of the aorta as a cause of positive FDG PET/CT. Clin Nucl Med 2007;32(9):729–31.

43. Tezuka D, Haraguchi G, Ishihara T, et al. Role of FDG PET-CT in Takayasu arteritis: sensitive detection of recurrences. JACC Cardiovasc Imaging 2012;5(4): 422–9.

44. Mehta NN, Yu Y, Saboury B, et al. Systemic and vascular inflammation in patients with moderate to severe psoriasis as measured by [18F]-fluorodeoxyglucose positron emission tomography-computed tomography (FDG-PET/CT): a pilot study. Arch Dermatol 2011;147(9):1031–9.

45. Rose S, Sheth NH, Baker JF, et al. A comparison of vascular inflammation in psoriasis, rheumatoid arthritis, and healthy subjects by FDG-PET/CT: a pilot study. Am J Cardiovasc Dis 2013;3(4):273–8.

46. Naik HB, Natarajan B, Stansky E, et al. Severity of psoriasis associates with aortic vascular inflammation detected by FDG PET/CT and neutrophil activation in a prospective observational study. Arterioscler Thromb Vasc Biol 2015;35(12):2667–76.

47. Powers WJ, Zazulia AR. PET in cerebrovascular disease. PET Clin 2010;5(1):83106.

48. Sah BR, Husmann L, Mayer D, et al. Diagnostic performance of 18F-FDG-PET/CT in vascular graft infections. Eur J Vasc Endovasc Surg 2015;49(4): 455–64.

49. Husmann L, Sah BR, Scherrer A, et al. (1)(8)F-FDG PET/CT for therapy control in vascular graft infections: a first feasibility study. J Nucl Med 2015; 56(7):1024–9.

50. Makis W, Stern J. Chronic vascular graft infection with fistula to bone causing vertebral osteomyelitis, imaged with F-18 FDG PET/CT. Clin Nucl Med 2010;35(10):794–6.

51. Hagenaars JC, Wever PC, Vlake AW, et al. Value of 18F-FDG PET/CT in diagnosing chronic Q fever in patients with central vascular disease. Neth J Med 2016;74(7):301–8.

52. Hsiao E, Laury A, Rybicki FJ, et al. Images in vascular medicine. Metastatic aortic intimal sarcoma: the use of PET/CT in diagnosing and staging. Vasc Med 2011;16(1):81–2.

53. von Falck C, Meyer B, Fegbeutel C, et al. Imaging features of primary sarcomas of the great vessels in CT, MRI and PET/CT: a single-center experience. BMC Med Imaging 2013;13:25.

54. Naswa N, Kumar R, Bal C, et al. Vascular thrombosis as a cause of abdominal pain in a patient with neuroendocrine carcinoma of pancreas: findings on (68) Ga-DOTANOC PET/CT. Indian J Nucl Med 2012; 27(1):35–7.

55. Malik D, Basher R, Vadi S, et al. Cardiac metastasis from lung cancer mimicking as perfusion defect on N-13 ammonia and FDG myocardial viability PET/CT scan. J Nucl Cardiol 2016. http://dx.doi.org/10.1007/s12350-016-0609-x.

PET/Computed Tomography and Precision Medicine
Musculoskeletal Sarcoma

Asha Kandathil, MD[a],*, Rathan M. Subramaniam, MD, PhD, MPH[a,b,c,d,e,f]

KEYWORDS

- Soft tissue sarcoma • Skeletal sarcoma • Molecular targeted therapy • PET • PET/CT

KEY POINTS

- The American College of Radiology appropriateness criteria propose the use of ^{18}F-fluorodeoxyglucose (FDG) PET as a primary diagnostic tool for detection and surveillance of metastases in patients with high-grade musculoskeletal tumors.
- National Comprehensive Cancer Network (NCCN) guidelines and imaging guidelines from the Children's Oncology Group Bone Tumor Committee recommend radionuclide bone scan and/or PET/CT scan for whole-body staging for osteosarcoma and Ewing sarcoma.
- NCCN recommends PET/computed tomography (CT) for clarification of ambiguous findings on CT or MR imaging during treatment response assessment in patients with gastrointestinal stromal tumors. If necessary, PET/CT may be used to assess early response to Imatinib after 2 to 4 weeks of therapy.
- ^{18}F-FDG PET/CT is useful in posttreatment evaluation, particularly after molecular targeted therapies. Pretherapy and posttherapy ^{18}F-FDG PET/CT metabolic parameters are reliable predictors of survival.
- ^{18}F-FDG PET/CT is valuable in evaluating tumor recurrence.

INTRODUCTION

Bone and soft tissue sarcomas, a heterogeneous group of malignant mesenchymal tumors, account for more than 20% of all pediatric solid malignant cancers and less than 1% of all adult solid malignant cancers. The vast majority are soft tissue sarcomas, with bone sarcomas accounting for about 10% of sarcomas.[1] Soft tissue sarcomas have a 5-year relative survival rate of approximately 65%.[2] Patients with bone sarcoma have a better outcome than patients with high-grade soft tissue sarcoma, and patients with extremity soft tissue sarcomas have better outcome compared with those in truncal sites. In 2017, it is estimated that approximately 12,390 new soft tissue sarcomas will be diagnosed (6890 cases in men and 5500

a Department of Radiology, The University of Texas Southwestern Medical Center, 5323 Harry Hines Boulevard, Dallas, TX 75390-8896, USA; b The Russell H. Morgan Department of Radiology and Radiological Sciences, The Johns Hopkins University School of Medicine, 601 North Caroline Street, Baltimore, MD 21287, USA; c Department of Clinical Sciences, The University of Texas Southwestern Medical Center, 5323 Harry Hines Boulevard, Dallas, TX 75390-8896, USA; d Department of Biomedical Engineering, The University of Texas Southwestern Medical Center, 5323 Harry Hines Boulevard, Dallas, TX 75390-8896, USA; e Department of Nuclear Medicine, Advanced Imaging Research Center, The University of Texas Southwestern Medical Center, 5323 Harry Hines Boulevard, Dallas, TX 75390-8896, USA; f Department of Nuclear Medicine, Harold C. Simmons Comprehensive Cancer Center, The University of Texas Southwestern Medical Center, 5323 Harry Hines Boulevard, Dallas, TX 75390-8896, USA
* Corresponding author.
E-mail address: asha.kandathil@utsouthwestern.edu

PET Clin 12 (2017) 475–488
http://dx.doi.org/10.1016/j.cpet.2017.05.005
1556-8598/17/© 2017 Elsevier Inc. All rights reserved.

cases in women) and 3260 new cancer of the bones and joints will be diagnosed.[2]

Soft tissue sarcomas have varied genetic makeup, have more than 50 histologic subtypes, and are often associated with differing clinical and prognostic features.[3–5] These tumors, which arise in the muscle, fat, blood vessels, nerves, tendons, or synovium, include embryonal rhabdomyosarcoma in children, synovial sarcoma in young adults, and high-grade pleomorphic sarcoma, liposarcoma, and leiomyosarcoma in adults. Most are located in the extremities (most common in thigh) with a few in the chest wall and retroperitoneum. Gastrointestinal stromal tumors (GISTs) are the most common primary mesenchymal tumors of the gastrointestinal tract. Soft tissue sarcomas become more common with increasing age, and there is a slight male predominance.

MOLECULAR GENETICS

Various dysregulated molecular pathways, including vascular endothelial growth factor stimulation of angiogenesis (VEGF), platelet-derived growth factor (PDGF) activation of signaling pathways, and aberrant activation of mitogen-activated protein kinase (MAPK) signaling pathway, are implicated in the oncogenesis of soft tissue sarcoma.

Knowledge of the propensity of specific sarcoma subtypes for specific pathway alterations is critical for developing effective targeted therapy. Pazopanib, an anti-VEGF-targeted molecular therapy with antiangiogenic effects mediated by kinase inhibition, is US Food and Drug Administration approved for treatment of soft tissue sarcomas.[6] Olaratumab, a monoclonal antibody that prevents platelet-derived growth factor receptor-alpha (PDGFR-a) from binding with several ligands on cancer cells, is indicated for treatment of some patients with metastatic soft tissue sarcoma.[7]

GISTs show activating mutations in CD117 (*KIT*) (75%–80%) or platelet-derived growth factor receptor alpha (PDGFRa) (5%–10%), which serve as diagnostic and therapeutic targets. Imatinib mesylate, a c-KIT tyrosine kinase inhibitor (TKI), is approved for the treatment of advanced or metastatic GIST. Sunitinib, a vascular endothelial growth factor receptor (VEGFR) inhibitor, has beneficial effect in imatinib-resistant GISTs[8] (**Fig. 1**).

Soft Tissue Sarcomas

Diagnosis and grading
[18]F- fluorodeoxyglucose (FDG) PET/computed tomography (CT) combines anatomic data with functional and metabolic information. The anatomic detail provided by CT, such as tumor size and local aggressiveness, is complemented by the metabolic information that PET provides. PET/CT also provides a guide to biopsy of the most aggressive

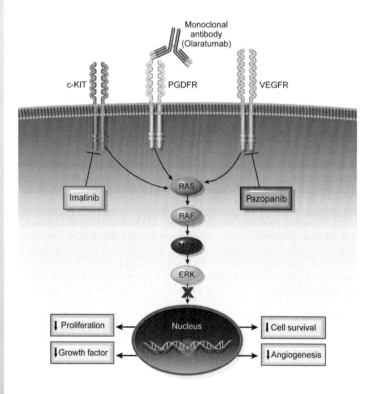

Fig. 1. Diagram of molecular genetics and molecular-targeted therapy in sarcoma. Activation of c-KIT, PDGFR, and VEGFR leads to downstream signaling through the PI3K and MAPK pathways promoting malignancies. Targeted therapeutic agents block these receptors and downstream signaling, resulting in decreased cell-cycle progression, cell survival, and angiogenesis.

portion of the lesion and may identify distant metastases.

A 2016 meta-analysis of the role of ^{18}F-FDG PET and ^{18}F-FDG PET/CT in the diagnosis of soft tissue musculoskeletal malignancies by Etchebehere and colleagues[9] showed that ^{18}F-FDG PET/CT and dedicated PET are both highly accurate in the diagnosis of musculoskeletal soft tissue lesions. The investigators included 14 articles from 1996 to March 2015 composed of 755 patients with 757 soft tissue lesions, comparing the diagnostic accuracy of ^{18}F-FDG PET/CT or dedicated PET with histopathology in patients with musculoskeletal soft tissue lesions. The ^{18}F-FDG PET/CT mean sensitivity, specificity, accuracy, positive predictive value, and negative predictive value for diagnosing musculoskeletal soft tissue lesions were 96%, 77%, 88%, 86%, and 90%, respectively. The optimal maximum standard uptake value (SUV_{max}) threshold value from 10 studies that best separated benign from malignant musculoskeletal lesions was 2.4. Folpe and colleagues[10] found that there was a significant overlap in SUV values between low-grade (grade 1) and high-grade (grades 2 and 3) sarcomas as well as high FDG uptake in benign tumors such as giant cell tumor of bone. When an SUV value of greater than 7.5 was used as cutoff, 93% of tumors were high-grade sarcomas; however, 52% of high-grade tumors had SUVmax of less than 7.5. Folpe and colleagues suggest that high SUV, indicative

of high metabolic rates, may be seen in high-grade sarcomas, highly cellular and proliferative tumors such as giant cell tumor of bone, and in slowly growing tumors with abundant matrix production such as fibromatoses.

Histopathologic grading done on a well-targeted biopsy determines management and prognosis of patients with soft tissue sarcoma. Varying FDG uptake by the tumor reflects intratumoral heterogeneity with areas of high SUV representing higher histologic grade, which can be targeted for biopsy (**Fig. 2**). Eary and colleagues[11] showed that tumor FDG uptake expressed as SUV_{max} had a high level of correlation with tumor grade of soft tissue sarcomas. In a retrospective evaluation of 238 consecutive patients with known soft tissue or osseous sarcoma who underwent ^{18}F-FDG PET/CT for initial staging or assessment of recurrence, Rakheja and colleagues[12] found a statistically significant correlation between the mitotic count and the SUV_{max} as well as between the presence of tumor necrosis and SUV_{max}. The median SUV_{max} values of sarcomas with mitotic counts of less than 2.00 (per 10 high-power fields) was 5.0, and those with mitotic counts of 16.25 or greater was 13.0.

Staging

Bone and soft tissue sarcomas predominantly metastasize to the lungs,[13] and CT scan of the chest is the examination of choice for detection of lung metastatic disease. Retroperitoneal and

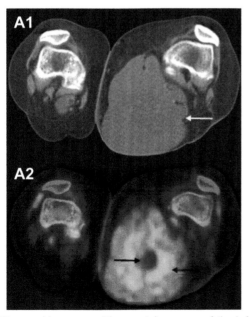
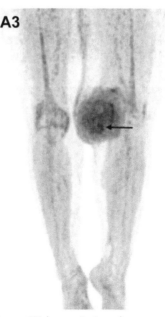

Fig. 2. A 53-year-old woman with synovial sarcoma of the left knee. CT demonstrates a homogenous soft tissue mass (*arrow*, *A1*) in the posteromedial aspect of the knee. On ^{18}F-FDG PET/CT, there is heterogeneous FDG uptake and central hypometabolic region representing necrosis (*arrows*, *A2*). Targeted biopsy from the most metabolically active portion of the tumor (*arrow*, *A3*) is likely to yield the highest tumor grade.

visceral sarcomas may spread hematogenously to the liver, and metastases to the retroperitoneum, spine, and paraspinous soft tissues are seen with myxoid liposarcomas. Synovial sarcoma, rhabdomyosarcoma, angiosarcoma, clear cell sarcoma, and epithelioid sarcoma have a predilection for spread to locoregional lymph nodes[14] (Fig. 3).

Tateishi and colleagues[15] demonstrated that staging accuracy improved when interpretations were based on combined PET/CT and conventional imaging, such as contrast-enhanced CT, bone scan, and MR imaging of the primary site. Combined PET/CT and conventional imaging resulted in correct N staging in 97% of patients and M staging in 93% of patients. In a study by Roberge and colleagues[16] on 109 patients with mostly intermediate- or high-grade soft tissue sarcomas, PET scans were normal for distant disease in 91/109 cases with a negative predictive value of 89%. The positive predictive value was 79%, and 5 patients were upstaged by FDG PET (4.5%). Volker and colleagues[17] compared PET/CT with conventional imaging (ultrasound, CT, MR imaging, and bone scintigraphy) in a prospective multicenter study of 46 pediatric patients with histologically proven sarcoma. They showed that PET/CT had a higher sensitivity (100%, 95%, and 89%, respectively) compared with conventional imaging modalities (100%, 25%, and 57%, respectively) in detection of primary tumors, lymph node involvement, and bone lesions. However, CT was superior to ^{18}F-FDG PET for the detection of lung metastases (sensitivity: 100% vs 25%, respectively). Khiewvan and colleagues[18] demonstrated that PET/CT had high accuracy of 88% in staging and 100% sensitivity in detecting local recurrence and distant metastases at restaging of patients with malignant peripheral nerve sheath tumor.

The American College of Radiology (ACR) appropriateness criteria, which are imaging guidelines set forth by the ACR, proposes the use of ^{18}F-FDG PET as a primary diagnostic tool for detection and surveillance of metastases, in patients with high-grade musculoskeletal tumors.[19]

Prognostication

Baseline tumor SUV_{max} has been shown to be an independent predictor of overall survival. In a study of 209 patients with soft tissue sarcomas, Eary and colleagues[20] showed that patients whose tumor SUV_{max} values are greater than the median SUV_{max} of 6.0 had a poorer prognosis than those whose tumor SUV_{max} values were less than 6.

Skamene and colleagues[21] demonstrated that bone and soft tissue sarcomas with an SUVmax of ≥ 10.3 had a 2-fold risk of progression and 2.4 times greater risk of death. A recent meta-analysis of 6 studies by Kubo and colleagues[22] of the prognostic significance of ^{18}F-FDG PET at diagnosis in patients with soft tissue sarcoma and bone sarcoma indicates that high SUV_{max} predicts significantly shorter overall survival periods than low SUV_{max}.

Therapy monitoring

Surgical resection remains the principal therapeutic modality in soft tissue sarcoma. Neoadjuvant or adjuvant chemotherapy and radiotherapy are given based on the histologic subtype. Chemotherapy with doxorubicin either as monotherapy or in combination with ifosfamide is the standard

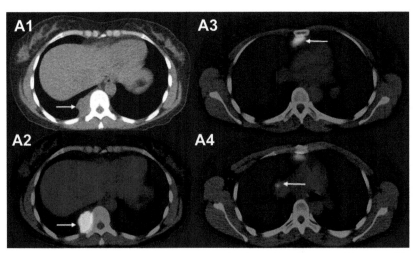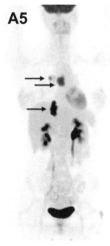

Fig. 3. A 30-year-old woman with stage IV (T2N1M1a) pulmonary blastoma. ^{18}F-FDG PET/CT demonstrates an FDG-avid right lower lobe mass (*arrow*, *A1*, *A2*, *A5*), right upper nodule (*arrow*, *A3*, *A5*), and right hilar node (*arrow*, *A4*, *A5*).

first-line treatment in metastatic soft tissue sarcomas.[23] Molecular targeted therapies such as Pazopanib and Olaratumab are indicated to treat certain subtypes of soft tissue sarcomas.

Benz and colleagues[24] prospectively studied the role of FDG PET/CT before (baseline), after the first cycle (early follow-up), and after completion of neoadjuvant therapy (late follow-up) in predicting histopathologic treatment response in high-grade soft tissue sarcomas. A 35% reduction in tumor FDG uptake at early follow-up was found to be a sensitive predictor of histopathologic tumor response. At late follow-up, a 60% decrease in tumor FDG uptake had a sensitivity of 75% and specificity of 68% in differentiating histopathologic responders and nonresponders.

^{18}F-FDG PET/CT has been prospectively validated as a strong predictor of histopathological response and progression-free survival, for both neoadjuvant and palliative chemotherapy in patients with soft tissue sarcomas. In a study by Eary and colleagues,[25] percentage reduction between the pretherapy and midtherapy SUVmax was a strong predictor of patient outcome. They suggest that a patient who has a high pretherapy SUV_{max} and little change in tumor uptake with therapy may consider discontinuing that line of treatment, whereas a patient with a high pretherapy SUV_{max} but a high SUV difference could be encouraged to continue treatment, because better survival could be predicted. In a study evaluating the histopathologic response to neoadjuvant therapy in high-grade soft tissue sarcomas, Evilevitch and colleagues[26] demonstrated that reduction in tumor FDG uptake, 5 to 15 days after treatment, was significantly greater in histopathologic responders than in nonresponders, whereas no significant differences were found for tumor size. Using a 60% decrease in tumor FDG uptake as a threshold resulted in a sensitivity of 100% and a specificity of 71% for assessment of histopathologic response, whereas tumor size reduction by Response Evaluation Criteria in Solid Tumors criteria showed a sensitivity of 25% and a specificity of 100%. With the advent of new molecular drugs such as Olaratumab, value of PET/CT in posttreatment response assessment is still evolving. Tissue markers and imaging modalities are needed to obtain specific information at molecular levels.

Tumor recurrence

^{18}F-FDG PET/CT is valuable in evaluating tumor recurrence. Al-Ibraheem and colleagues[27] demonstrated that ^{18}F-FDG PET/CT has greater diagnostic accuracy in the detection of recurrent bone or soft tissue sarcoma compared with contrast-enhanced CT alone, with sensitivity and

specificity of 83% and 100%. On retrospectively reviewing the images of 33 FDG PET scans, comparing the results with surgical pathology or clinical follow-up for at least 6 months, Johnson and colleagues[28] found that FDG PET detected all 25 cases of local and distant recurrences with 100% sensitivity. Dancheva and colleagues[29] evaluated 15 patients with suspected local sarcoma recurrence with 60-minute and 120-minute dual-time FDG PET-CT. Increase in SUVmax with percentage change over time per lesion (% DSUV) >10% in the delayed scan was considered indicative of recurrent malignancy. They found that in high-grade sarcomas dual-time imaging was more sensitive and accurate in identifying local tumor recurrence; however, there was limited benefit in low-grade sarcomas.

Gastrointestinal Stromal Tumors

GISTs are treated by surgical removal. Neoadjuvant or adjuvant molecularly targeted therapy, with imatinib mesylate, reduces the tumor burden and frequency of disease recurrence.[30] TKIs currently approved to treat metastatic GIST include imatinib, sunitinib, and regorafenib.[8]

Because functional and biochemical changes in a tumor in response to molecular targeted therapy precede morphologic changes, FDG PET demonstrates metabolic response before change in size is evident on cross-sectional imaging (Fig. 4). Metabolic response on [18]FDG PET has been observed as early as 24 hours after a single dose of imatinib and a significant change in SUV_{max} to less than 2.5 and/or a greater than 25% decrease in SUV_{max} relative to baseline can be seen within 1 month of starting imatinib therapy in all GIST patients responding to the drug.[31] Treglia and colleagues[32] did a systematic review of 19 studies evaluating the role of [18]FDG PET/CT in assessing treatment response to imatinib or other drugs in GISTs. They found that ^{18}F-FDG PET is useful for early assessment of treatment response, a valuable method for posttherapy follow-up and a good predictor of clinical outcome. In a study, evaluating the value of ^{18}F-FDG PET/CT in assessing early response of soft tissue sarcomas to therapy with imatinib mesylate, Stroobants and colleagues[33] found that a complete metabolic response was achieved within 1 week in most of the responding patients, including all GISTs, and preceded CT response by several weeks. In a 2016 meta-analysis of 21 articles by Hassanzadeh-Rad and colleagues,[34] the pooled sensitivity of ^{18}F-FDG PET/CT in evaluation of response to treatment of GIST was 90% and specificity was 62%. ^{18}F-FDG PET/CT is also useful in resolving ambiguous findings on contrast-enhanced CT, such as

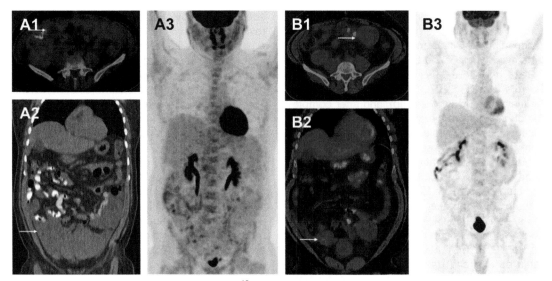

Fig. 4. A 46-year-old man with metastatic GIST. ^{18}F-FDG PET/CT obtained after a few cycles of imatinib demonstrates residual peritoneal masses (*arrow, A2*) without increased FDG uptake (*arrow, A1, A3*), indicating good metabolic response. Three-year follow-up ^{18}F-FDG PET/CT demonstrates decrease in size and extent of peritoneal disease with continued metabolic response (*arrow, B1, B2, B3*).

posttreatment intratumoral hemorrhage, which can mimic tumor recurrence on CT.

Several studies have found that SUV_{max} on preoperative ^{18}F-FDG PET/CT may predict malignant potential of GIST.[35–37] In a study on 26 patients with GIST by Park and colleagues[35] using a cutoff value for SUV_{max} of 3.94, the sensitivity and specificity for predicting the risk of malignancy were 85.7% and 94.7%, respectively. The SUV_{max} of ^{18}F-FDG PET/CT was associated with Ki-67 index, tumor size, mitotic count, and National Institutes of Health risk classification. However, in a study by Choi and colleagues,[38] 21% of lesions ranging in size from 1.0 to 4.7 cm were not FDG avid before treatment, precluding its application in posttreatment monitoring.

As most GISTs tend to recur within the first 3 to 5 years, intense follow-up is required during this period. Most patients develop resistance to molecular targeted therapy with imatinib, which can be either primary resistance, defined as disease progression in the first 6 months of treatment, or secondary resistance, with tumor progression after initial good response for more than 6 months.[8] Lack of metabolic response on ^{18}F-FDG PET/CT indicates primary resistance to the drug, whereas reemergence of metabolic activity within tumor sites after a period of therapeutic response indicates secondary resistance to the drug (**Fig. 5**). A characteristic CT pattern of recurrence is "nodule-within-cyst" appearance seen as new enhancing tumor nodules in a nonenhancing cystic mass. Such patients may benefit from other molecular targeted therapy, as sunitinib and regorafenib. When imatinib

was stopped in patients with refractory GIST, marked increase in FDG uptake within the tumor, known as the flare phenomenon, suggests that portions of the tumor were still responding to imatinib, whereas other parts had developed resistance.[39]

Prior and colleagues[40] evaluated treatment response on ^{18}F-FDG PET/CT in 23 patients treated with sunitinib after imatinib failure. They found that ^{18}F-FDG PET/CT after 4 weeks of treatment with sunitinib is useful for early assessment of treatment response and for the prediction of clinical outcome. In their study, when the SUV was less than 8 g/mL, median progression-free survival was 29 weeks as compared with 4 weeks for SUV of 8 g/mL or greater.

During posttreatment response assessment in patients with GIST, the National Comprehensive Cancer Network (NCCN) recommends use of PET/CT for clarification of ambiguous findings on CT or MR imaging. If necessary, PET/CT may be used to assess early response to Imitanib after 2 to 4 weeks of therapy.[41]

Skeletal Sarcoma

Other than multiple myeloma, osteosarcoma is the most common malignant primary bone tumor, accounting for 30% of tumors. Osteosarcomas have peak incidence in adolescents. In patients greater than 60 years of age, they arise as secondary tumors in Paget disease or in previously irradiated tissue. Chondrosarcoma is the second most common malignant primary tumor of bone. Ewing sarcoma accounts for approximately 6% of all

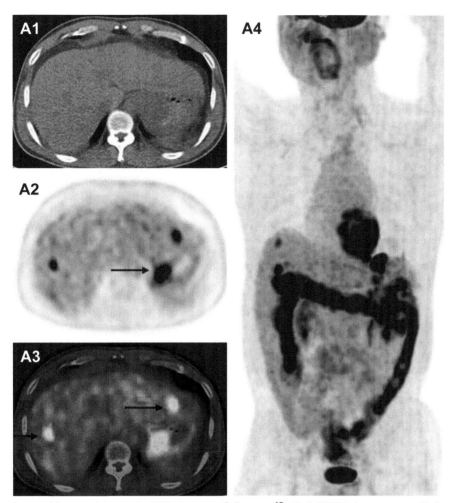

Fig. 5. A 45-year-old man with gastric GIST. One-year follow-up ^{18}F-FDG PET/CT demonstrates FDG-avid gastric tumor (*arrow, A1, A2*) and metabolically active liver metastases (*arrow, A3, A4*).

primary malignant bone tumors, and malignant fibrous histiocytoma accounts for less than 1% of primary bone sarcomas.[3] Management of musculoskeletal malignancies is based on accurate assessment of the extent of primary tumor and presence of metastatic disease.[42] The 5-year survival of patients with osteosarcoma or Ewing sarcoma is 65% to 70% with localized disease compared with only 20% for those with metastatic disease.[43] Patients with suspected bone tumor are initially evaluated with plain radiography of the region of interest, followed by MR imaging of the whole extremity. Diagnosis is confirmed by biopsy.[44] A bone scan or PET scan is recommended for staging to detect metastatic bone and soft tissue disease.[45] Because more than 75% of metastases involve the lungs, all patients with bone sarcoma should receive a thin-section CT scan of the chest.

NCCN guidelines and imaging guidelines from the Children's Oncology Group Bone Tumor Committee for both osteosarcoma and Ewing sarcoma recommend radionuclide bone scan and/or PET scan for whole-body staging.[45] Several studies have demonstrated the prognostic value of pretreatment FDG PET/CT, which offers the potential for patients at high risk for relapse or metastases to be considered for more aggressive systemic chemotherapy than low- or intermediate-risk patients (**Fig. 6**).

Tumor necrosis induced by neoadjuvant chemotherapy is one of the most powerful prognostic indicators of survival in patients with osteosarcoma and Ewing sarcoma. FDG PET has been found to be a noninvasive surrogate of response to neoadjuvant chemotherapy in monitoring treatment response with potential to individualize and optimize patient therapy.

Osteosarcoma

Diagnosis and staging In a study by Costelloe and colleagues,[46] a high prechemotherapy SUV$_{max}$ in

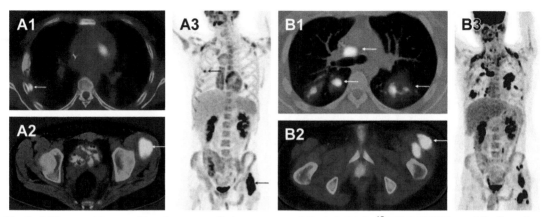

Fig. 6. A 22-year-old man with extraosseous Ewing sarcoma of the left thigh. ^{18}F-FDG PET/CT scan (*A*) after a few cycles of chemotherapy demonstrates intense FDG uptake in the left thigh mass (*arrow, A2, A3*) and a right pleural lesion (*arrow, A1, A3*). One-year follow-up ^{18}F-FDG PET/CT scan (*B*) demonstrates FDG-avid metastatic pulmonary nodules, mediastinal nodes (*arrows, B1, B3*), and local tumor recurrence (*arrow, B2, B3*).

patients with osteosarcoma correlated with worse progression-free survival, and a high postchemotherapy SUV$_{max}$ correlated with both worse progression-free survival and poor overall survival. Byun and colleagues[47] retrospectively reviewed ^{18}F-FDG PET and bone scan in 206 patients with osteosarcoma. For detection of bone metastases, the sensitivity, specificity, and diagnostic accuracy for PET/CT were 95%, 98%, and 98%, respectively, and 76%, 97%, and 96%, respectively, for bone scan. Quartuccio and colleagues[48] reviewed 13 studies on the diagnostic accuracy of ^{18}F-FDG PET or PET/CT in patients with different types of sarcomas, including some patients with osteosarcoma. They concluded that FDG PET and PET/CT had high diagnostic performance and seemed to be superior to bone scintigraphy and conventional imaging methods in detecting bone metastases; however, thin-section chest CT scan was superior to ^{18}F-FDG PET in detecting pulmonary metastases from osteosarcoma. In a study by London and colleagues,[49] the accuracy of ^{18}F-FDG PET was compared with conventional imaging modalities, including ultrasound, CT, MR imaging, and bone scintigraphy in children with metastatic osteosarcoma and Ewing sarcoma. ^{18}F-FDG PET detected distant metastases with greater sensitivity and specificity (98% and 97%, respectively) compared with conventional imaging modalities (83% and 78%, respectively). However, CT was again superior to ^{18}F-FDG PET for the detection of lung metastases.

Therapy monitoring FDG PET imaging has evolved as a noninvasive method to assess response to neoadjuvant chemotherapy.

In a 2012 meta-analysis of 8 studies by Hongtao and colleagues[50] to evaluate the value of ^{18}F-FDG PET/CT in the assessment of histologic response to neoadjuvant chemotherapy in patients with osteosarcomas, SUV$_{max}$ after treatment ≤2.5 and ratio of posttreatment and pretreatment SUV$_{max}$ ≤0.5 were found to be predictive of histologic response to chemotherapy. In a study on 40 patients with extremity osteosarcoma who received neoadjuvant and adjuvant chemotherapy, Hawkins and colleagues[51] found that median SUV value less than 2.5 in the ^{18}F-FDG PET/CT following neoadjuvant chemotherapy was associated with improved progression-free survival. Bajpai and colleagues[52] prospectively evaluated 31 osteosarcoma patients with ^{18}F-FDG PET/CT before and after 3 cycles of neoadjuvant chemotherapy, comparing morphologic and metabolic parameters to postsurgical histopathologic analysis. They found that patients with pretreatment tumor volume ≤300 mL and ratio of posttreatment and pretreatment SUV$_{max}$ ≤0.48 had good histologic response.

Ye and colleagues[53] evaluated the role of SUV$_{max}$ of tumor and tumor-to-background ratio (TBR) before (TBR1) and after chemotherapy (TBR2) in patients with osteosarcoma. TBR was calculated by drawing an identical region of interest over the tumor and the contralateral normal limb or pelvis. Comparison was made to histologically assessed tumor necrosis. They found that in patients with favorable response, TBR2/TBR1 was less than 0.46 and greater than 0.49 in those with unfavorable responses.

In a prospective study of 31 patients with osteosarcoma, Byun and colleagues[54] evaluated the ability of dual-phase^{18} F-FDG PET/CT with both early (~60 minutes) and delayed (~150 minutes)

PET to predict the histologic response after neoadjuvant chemotherapy in osteosarcoma. They evaluated early/delayed SUV$_{max}$ change and early/delayed SUVmean change in both pretherapy and posttherapy scans. In the pretreatment scans, only early/delayed SUVmean change predicted good therapeutic response with the optimal criterion of less than 10%. Early/delayed SUV change of tumors significantly decreased after neoadjuvant chemotherapy. In a study on 31 patients with osteosarcoma and Ewing sarcoma, Choong and colleagues[55] demonstrated a 50% reduction in metabolic tumor volume (MTV) was found to be significantly associated with histologic response in osteosarcoma. Denecke and colleagues[56] found significant relationship between FDG uptake and tumor necrosis in osteosarcoma.

Tumor recurrence Limb-salvage surgery with tumor resection and endoprosthetic replacement is the standard treatment of extremity osteosarcoma. The presence of metallic artifacts limits evaluation for local recurrence with CT and MR imaging. Chronic periprosthetic inflammation will result in increased FDG uptake. Chang and colleagues[57] retrospectively reviewed 355 ^{18}F-FDG PET/CT scans in 109 extremity osteosarcoma patients to assess the ability of changes of increased ^{18}F-FDG uptake around the prosthesis to differentiate local recurrence from postsurgical change after tumor resection and endoprosthetic replacement. Nine patients (8%) had a local recurrence. SUVmax at 3 months (SUV1) and SUVmax at the time of local recurrence in patients with recurrence or at the last follow-up in others (SUV2) were compared. The combination of SUV2 greater than 4.6 and change in SUV greater than 75% was found to be a useful parameter for identifying local recurrence with sensitivity, specificity, and accuracy of 78%, 94%, 93% respectively.

Ewing sarcoma

The Ewing sarcoma family of tumors (ESFT) includes Ewing tumor of bone, extraosseous Ewing tumor, and peripheral primitive neuroectodermal tumor.[2]

Diagnosis and staging In a study by Gupta and colleagues[58] on 54 patients with ESFT, there was a statistically significant difference in mean SUV$_{max}$ of tumors with and without metastases at presentation, reflecting aggressive behavior. The mean SUV$_{max}$ in the primary tumor in patients without metastases was 6.84 and in those with metastases were 11.31.

In a meta-analysis of 5 studies, Treglia and colleagues[59] showed that ^{18}F-FDG PET and PET/CT have high sensitivity of 96% and high specificity

of 92% in the detection of ESFT. They found that ^{18}F-FDG PET/CT is a valuable method in staging of Ewing sarcoma and in detecting recurrences, compared with other imaging modalities such as bone scan and whole body MR imaging. Spiral CT was found to be more sensitive for detection of small lung metastases.

In a study of 24 patients with suspected Ewing tumor, Györke and colleagues[60] found that the sensitivity and specificity of ^{18}F-FDG PET/CT for detection of primary tumor and/or its metastases were 96% and 78%, respectively. ^{18}F-FDG PET/CT had lower sensitivity for detection of smaller lesions, and there was overlap of SUV mean between malignant and benign lesions. In true-positive cases, the mean SUV was 4.54 ± 2.79.

^{18}F-FDG PET/CT is more sensitive and specific than bone scan for detecting osseous metastases: in a study of 38 patients who had primary Ewing sarcoma, FDG PET showed higher accuracy (97% vs 82%), sensitivity (100% vs 68%), and specificity (96% vs 87%) than bone scan.[61]

Therapy monitoring Many studies have found a significant correlation between change in metabolic activity of the primary tumor and histopathological response after neoadjuvant chemotherapy.

In a study evaluating the response of Ewing sarcoma family of tumors to neoadjuvant chemotherapy, Hawkins and colleagues[62] found that posttreatment ^{18}F-FDG PET/CT SUVmax less than 2.5 is predictive of progression-free survival, independent of initial disease stage. Palmerini and colleagues[63] evaluated the role of ^{18}F-FDG PET/CT in 77 patients (45 with Ewing sarcoma and 32 with osteosarcoma) treated with neoadjuvant chemotherapy. They showed an association between pretreatment SUV$_{max}$ and histologic/radiological response in patients with osteosarcoma and in those with Ewing sarcoma. A study on 54 patients with ESFT[58] also found that percentage change in SUV$_{max}$ before and after 4 cycles of neoadjuvant therapy correlated well with percentage necrosis on histopathological examination. Choong and colleagues[55] demonstrated that a 90% reduction in MTV was associated with histologic response in Ewing's sarcoma (**Fig. 7**)

Tumor recurrence In a study in 19 children with sarcoma (9 Ewing sarcoma, 3 osteogenic sarcoma, 7 rhabdomyosarcoma) by Arush and colleagues,[64] findings on FDG PET CT were compared with surgical pathology or clinical follow-up for at least 3 months. FDG PET CT was positive in all 7 patients with tumor recurrence at the primary site and in 77% of those with distant metastases. In a retrospective analysis by

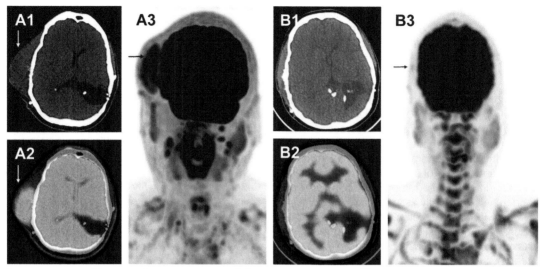

Fig. 7. A 23-year-old man with Ewing sarcoma of the scalp. Initial staging ^{18}F-FDG PET/CT demonstrates an FDG-avid soft tissue mass (*arrow, A1, A2, A3*) in the right scalp. Postneoadjuvant ^{18}F-FDG PET/CT demonstrates good anatomic and metabolic response (*arrow, B1, B2, B3*).

Franzius and colleagues,[61] FDG PET/CT identified local recurrence in 6 patients with osteosarcoma and 21 patients with Ewing sarcomas when compared with histopathological analysis and/or the clinical and imaging follow-up (**Fig. 8**).

CHONDROSARCOMA

^{18}F-FDG PET/CT may be of value in noninvasively assessing tumor grade, identifying otherwise occult metastatic disease, and differentiating recurrent tumor from postoperative change in patients with chondrosarcoma.

Lee and colleagues[65] evaluated the diagnostic value and limitations of ^{18}F-FDG PET/CT for cartilaginous tumors of bone. They correlated SUV_{max} of 35 biopsy-proven cartilaginous tumors with histopathologic grade, tumor size, recurrence, and metastasis. There was no significant difference in SUV_{max} between benign cartilage tumors and grade 1 chondrosarcomas; however, there was a significant difference between the low-grade and high-grade chondrosarcomas. SUV_{max} of 2.3 or greater had a positive predictive value of 82% and negative predictive value of 96% for grade 2 or 3 chondrosarcomas. Higher SUV_{max} of the

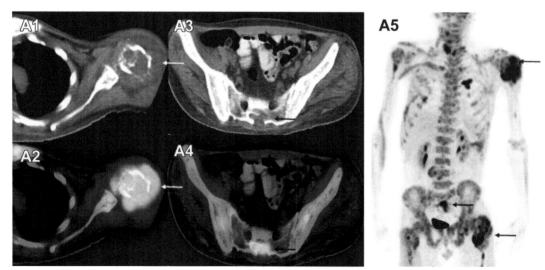

Fig. 8. A 43-year-old man 1-year postresection of sacral Ewing sarcoma. ^{18}F-FDG PET/CT demonstrates local tumor recurrence (*arrow, A3, A4, A5*) and bone metastases (*arrow, A1, A2, A5*).

primary tumor was associated with metastasis, but not tumor recurrence. Jesus-Garcia and colleagues[66] evaluated the role of ^{18}F-FDG PET/CT in differentiating chondroma and chondrosarcoma. They found 1 chondrosarcoma among the 17 patients with $SUV_{max} \leq 2.0$, and 18 chondrosarcomas and 1 chondroma among the 19 patients with SUV_{max} greater than 2.0. The investigators suggest that SUV_{max} between 2.0 and 2.2 would be a range area between chondroma and chondrosarcoma, and this range can be of value, in conjunction with other imaging modalities such as MR imaging, in deciding the best treatment of patients with cartilaginous lesions in long bones.

Purandare and colleagues[67] retrospectively evaluated the role of ^{18}F-FDG PET/CT in predicting sarcomatous transformation in 12 patients with osteochondromas. There was low-grade FDG uptake (SUV 0.8–1.3) in 4 patients with benign lesions, moderate to high FDG uptake in 7 patients with histopathological evidence of a sarcomatous transformation to grade 2 chondrosarcoma (SUV 3.3–6.9), and high uptake in 1 patient with a dedifferentiated chondrosarcoma (SUV 11.4).

Brenner and colleagues[68] evaluated the role of ^{18}F-FDG PET/CT for grading and prediction of outcome in chondrosarcoma patients. A combination of SUV_{max} and histopathologic tumor grade was found to have high sensitivity and specificity for identification of patients at high risk for relapse. A cutoff of 4 for SUV_{max} had sensitivity, specificity, and positive and negative predictive values of 90%, 76%, 64%, and 94%, respectively, for relapse.

NOVEL TRACERS
Role of ^{18}F-Fluorothymidine PET in Bone and Soft Tissue Sarcomas

PET using the radiotracer ^{18}F-fluorothymidine (FLT) can image tumor proliferation as a function of thymidine salvage pathway utilization with FLT uptake shown to correlate with the Ki-67 score. Osgood and colleagues[69] suggest that ^{18}F-FLT PET could be used as a novel diagnostic imaging approach for Ewing sarcoma because it reflects Ewing sarcoma-FLI1 activity in Ewing sarcoma cells. Cobben and colleagues[70] showed that ^{18}F-FLT PET, which reflects the proliferation activity of tissues, is taken up by soft tissue sarcomas and has the potential to differentiate between low-grade and high-grade soft tissue sarcomas. Benz and colleagues[71] evaluated the value of ^{18}F-FLT PET/CT, in assessment of tumor viability and proliferation in patients with soft tissue sarcomas who are treated with neoadjuvant therapy. They found that ^{18}F-FLT PET/CT imaging does not reliably predict histopathological response to neoadjuvant therapy.

SUMMARY

^{18}F-FDG PET/CT has been increasingly recognized as a useful adjunct to conventional imaging with radiography, CT, MR imaging, and bone scan in patients with bone and soft tissue sarcomas. It is indicated in staging of patients with high-grade sarcomas, detecting metastases, and guiding biopsy to the most aggressive portion of the tumor. It has an important role in posttreatment response assessment, particularly in evaluation of molecular targeted therapies, which induce metabolic change before structural change. During treatment response assessment in patients with GIST ^{18}F-FDG PET/CT is indicated for clarification of ambiguous findings on CT or MR imaging. ^{18}F-FDG PET/CT is valuable in detection of local tumor recurrence, particularly in patients with orthopedic hardware that limits evaluation with MR imaging or CT.

REFERENCES

1. Burningham Z, Hashibe M, Spector L, et al. The epidemiology of sarcoma. Clin Sarcoma Res 2012;2:14.
2. Available at: https://www.cancer.gov. Accessed June 27, 2017.
3. Available at: http://www.cancernetwork.com. Accessed June 27, 2017.
4. Fletcher DM, Bridge JA, Hogendoorn P, et al. Tumors of soft tissue and bone: pathology and genetics. World Health Organization classification of tumors. Lyon (France): IARC Press; 2013.
5. Italiano A, Le Cesne A, Blay JY, et al. Patterns of care and outcome of patients (pts) with metastatic soft-tissue sarcoma (STS) according to histological subtype and treatment setting: the METASTAR study. J Clin Oncol 2016;34(suppl) [abstract: 11014].
6. Sborov D, Chen JL. Targeted therapy in sarcomas other than GIST tumors. J Surg Oncol 2015;111:632–40.
7. Tap WD, Jones RL, Van Tine BA, et al. Olaratumab and doxorubicin versus doxorubicin alone for treatment of soft-tissue sarcoma: an open-label phase 1b and randomised phase 2 trial. Lancet 2016; 388(10043):488–97.
8. Tirumani SH, Jagannathan JP, Krajewski KM, et al. Imatinib and beyond in gastrointestinal stromal tumors: a radiologist's perspective. AJR Am J Roentgenol 2013;201:801–10.
9. Etchebehere EC, Hobbs BP, Milton DR, et al. Assessing the role of ^{18}F-FDG PET and ^{18}F-FDG PET/CT in the diagnosis of soft tissue musculoskeletal malignancies: a systematic review and meta-analysis. Eur J Nucl Med Mol Imaging 2016;43(5):860–70.

10. Folpe AL, Lyles RH, Sprouse JT, et al. (F-18) fluoro-deoxyglucose positron emission tomography as a predictor of pathologic grade and other prognostic variables in bone and soft tissue sarcoma. Clin Cancer Res 2000;6:1279–87.

11. Eary JF, Conrad EU, Bruckner JB, et al. Quantitative [F-18]fluorodeoxyglucose positron emission tomography in pre-treatment and grading of sarcoma. Clin Cancer Res 1998;4:1215–20.

12. Rakheja R, Makis W, Skamene S, et al. Correlating metabolic activity on 18F-FDG PET/CT with histopathologic characteristics of osseous and soft-tissue sarcomas: a retrospective review of 136 patients. AJR Am J Roentgenol 2012;198(6):1409–16.

13. Billingsley KG, Lewis JJ, Leung DH, et al. Multifactorial analysis of the survival of patients with distant metastasis arising from primary extremity sarcoma. Cancer 1999;85(2):389–95.

14. Riad S, Griffin AM, Liberman B, et al. Lymph node metastasis in soft tissue sarcoma in an extremity. Clin Orthop Relat Res 2004;(426):129–34.

15. Tateishi U, Yamaguchi U, Seki K, et al. Bone and soft-tissue sarcoma: preoperative staging with fluorine 18 fluorodeoxyglucose PET/CT and conventional imaging. Radiology 2007;245(3):839–47.

16. Roberge D, Vakilian S, Alabed YZ, et al. FDG PET/CT in initial staging of adult soft-tissue sarcoma. Sarcoma 2012;2012:960194.

17. Volker T, Denecke T, Steffen I, et al. Positron emission tomography for staging of pediatric sarcoma patients: results of a prospective multicenter trial. J Clin Oncol 2007;25:5435–41.

18. Khiewvan B, Macapinlac HA, Lev D, et al. The value of ^{18}F-FDG PET/CT in the management of malignant peripheral nerve sheath tumors. Eur J Nucl Med Mol Imaging 2014;41(9):1756–66.

19. Roberts CC, Kransdorf MJ, Beaman FD, et al. ACR appropriateness criteria follow-up of malignant or aggressive musculoskeletal tumors. J Am Coll Radiol 2016;13:389–400.

20. Eary JF, O'Sullivan F, Powitan Y, et al. Sarcoma tumor FDG uptake measured by PET and patient outcome: a retrospective analysis. Eur J Nucl Med Mol Imaging 2002;29(9):1149–54.

21. Skamene SR, Rakheja R, Dalhstrom KR, et al. Metabolic activity measured on PET/CT correlates with clinical outcomes in patients with limb and girdle sarcomas. J Surg Oncol 2014;109:410–4.

22. Kubo T, Furuta T, Johan MP, et al. Prognostic significance of (18)F-FDG PET at diagnosis in patients with soft tissue sarcoma and bone sarcoma; systematic review and meta-analysis. Eur J Cancer 2016;58:104–11.

23. Judson I, Verweij J, Gelderblom H, et al, for the European Organisation of Research and Treatment in Cancer Soft Tissue and Bone Sarcoma Group. Doxorubicin alone versus intensified doxorubicin plus ifosfamide for first line treatment of advanced or metastatic soft tissue sarcoma: a randomised controlled phase III trial. Lancet Oncol 2014;15:415–23.

24. Benz MR, Czernin J, Allen-Auerbach MS, et al. DG-PET/CT imaging predicts histopathologic treatment responses after the initial cycle of neoadjuvant chemotherapy in high-grade soft-tissue sarcomas. Clin Cancer Res 2009;15(8):2856–63.

25. Eary JF, Conrad EU, O'Sullivan J, et al. Sarcoma midtherapy [F-18]fluorodeoxyglucose positron emission tomography (FDG PET) and patient outcome. J Bone Joint Surg Am 2014;96(2):152–8.

26. Evilevitch V, Weber WA, Tap WD, et al. Reduction of glucose metabolic activity is more accurate than change in size at predicting histopathologic response to neoadjuvant therapy in high-grade soft-tissue sarcomas. Clin Cancer Res 2008;14(3):715–20.

27. Al-Ibraheem A, Buck AK, Benz MR, et al. 18F-Fluorodeoxyglucose positron emission tomography/computed tomography for the detection of recurrent bone and soft tissue sarcoma. Cancer 2013;119:1227–34.

28. Johnson GR, Zhuang H, Khan J, et al. Roles of positron emission tomography with fluorine-18-deoxyglucose in the detection of local recurrent and distant metastatic sarcoma. Clin Nucl Med 2003;28:815–20.

29. Dancheva Z, Bochev P, Chaushev B, et al. Dual-time point 18FDG-PET/CT imaging may be useful in assessing local recurrent disease in high grade bone and soft tissue sarcoma. Nucl Med Rev Cent East Eur 2016;19(1):22–7.

30. Rammohan A, Sathyanesan J, Rajendran K, et al. A gist of gastrointestinal stromal tumors: a review. World J Gastrointest Oncol 2013;5(6):102–12.

31. Van den Abbeele AD. The lessons of GIST—PET and PET/CT: a new paradigm for imaging. Oncologist 2008;13:8–13.

32. Treglia G, Mirk P, Stefanelli A, et al. 18F-fluorodeoxyglucose positron emission tomography in evaluating treatment response to imatinib or other drugs in gastrointestinal stromal tumors: a systematic review. Clin Imaging 2012;36:167–75.

33. Stroobants S, Goeminne J, Seegers M, et al. 18FDG-Positron emission tomography for the early prediction of response in advanced soft tissue sarcoma treated with imatinib mesylate (Glivec). Eur J Cancer 2003;39:2012–20.

34. Hassanzadeh-Rad A, Yousefifard M, Katal S, et al. The value of 18F-fluorodeoxyglucose positron emission tomography for prediction of treatment response in gastrointestinal stromal tumors: a systematic review and meta-analysis. J Gastroenterol Hepatol 2016;31:929–35.

35. Park JW, Cho CH, Jeong DS, et al. Role of F-fluoro-2-deoxyglucose positron emission tomography in

gastric GIST: predicting malignant potential pre-operatively. J Gastric Cancer 2011;11:173–9.

36. Kamiyama Y, Aihara R, Nakabayashi T, et al. 18F-fluorodeoxyglucose positron emission tomography: useful technique for predicting malignant potential of gastrointestinal stromal tumors. World J Surg 2005;29:1429–35.

37. Yoshikawa K, Shimada M, Kurita N, et al. The efficacy of PET–CT for predicting the malignant potential of gastrointestinal stromal tumors. Surg Today 2013;43:1162–7.

38. Choi H, Charnsangavej C, Faria S, et al. CT evaluation of the response of gastrointestinal stromal tumors after imatinib mesylate treatment: a quantitative analysis correlated with FDG PET findings. AJR Am J Roentgenol 2004;183: 1619–28.

39. Van Den Abbeele AD, Badawi RD, Manola J, et al. Effects of cessation of imatinib mesylate (IM) therapy in patients (pts) with IM refractory gastrointestinal stromal tumors (GIST) as visualized by FDGPET scanning [abstract]. J Clin Oncol 2004; 22(Suppl 1) [abstract: 3012].

40. Prior JO, Montemurro M, Orcurto MV, et al. Early prediction of response to sunitinib after imatinib failure by 18F-Fluorodeoxyglucose positron emission tomography in patients with gastrointestinal stromal tumor. J Clin Oncol 2009;27(3):439–45.

41. Demetri GD, von Mehren M, Antonescu CR, et al. NCCN Task Force Report: update on the management of patients with gastrointestinal stromal tumors. J Natl Compr Canc Netw 2010;8(Suppl 2):S1–41 [quiz: S42–4].

42. Purandare NC, Rangarajan V, EPurandare NC, et al. Emerging role of PET/CT in osteosarcoma. J Bone Soft Tissue Tumors 2016;2(1):19–21.

43. Quartuccio N, Fox J, Kuk D, et al. Pediatric bone sarcoma: diagnostic performance of 18F-FDG PET/CT versus conventional imaging for initial staging and follow-up. AJR Am J Roentgenol 2015;204(1): 153–60.

44. Durfee RA, Mohammed M, Luu HH. Review of osteosarcoma and current management. Rheumatol Ther 2016;3(2):221–43.

45. Sybil Biermann J, Adkins DR, Benjamin RS. Bone cancer NCCN clinical practice guidelines in oncology. J Natl Compr Canc Netw 2013;8(6):688–712.

46. Costelloe CM, Macapinlac HA, Madewell JE, et al. 18F-FDG PET/CT as an indicator of progression-free and overall survival in osteosarcoma. J Nucl Med 2009;50:340–7.

47. Byun GH, Kong CB, Lim I, et al. Comparison of (18) F-FDG PET/CT and (99 m)Tc-MDP bone scintigraphy for detection of bone metastasis in osteosarcoma. Skeletal Radiol 2013;42(12):1673–81.

48. Quartuccio N, Treglia G, Salsano M, et al. The role of fluorine-18-fluorodeoxyglucose positron emission tomography in staging and restaging of patients with osteosarcoma. Radiol Oncol 2013;47(2):97–102.

49. London K, Stege C, Cross S, et al. 18F-FDG PET/CT compared to conventional imaging modalities in pediatric primary bone tumors. Pediatr Radiol 2012;42:418–30.

50. Hongtao L, Hui Z, Bingshun W, et al. 18F-FDG positron emission tomography for the assessment of histological response to neoadjuvant chemotherapy in osteosarcomas: a meta-analysis. Surg Oncol 2012; 21(4):e165–70.

51. Hawkins DS, Conrad EU 3rd, Butrynski JE, et al. [F-18]-fluorodeoxy-D-glucose-positron emission tomography response is associated with outcome for extremity osteosarcoma in children and young adults. Cancer 2009;115(15):3519–25.

52. Bajpai J, Kumar R, Vishnubhatla S, et al. PET-CT in osteosarcoma for chemotherapy response evaluation: correlation with histological necrosis. J Nucl Med 2009;50(Suppl 2):582.

53. Ye Z, Zhu J, Tian M, et al. Response of osteogenic sarcoma to neoadjuvant therapy, evaluated by 18F-FDG-PET. Ann Nucl Med 2008;22(6):475–80.

54. Byun BH, Kim SH, Lim SM, et al. Prediction of response to neoadjuvant chemotherapy in osteosarcoma using dual-phase (18)F-FDG PET/CT. Eur Radiol 2015;25(7):2015–24.

55. Choong PF, Di Bella C, Gaston C, et al. F18-FDG PET response to neoadjuvant chemotherapy for Ewing's sarcoma and osteosarcoma are different. Orthopaedic Proc 2012;94-B(Supp XXXVIII):142.

56. Denecke T, Hundsdorfer P, Misch D, et al. Assessment of histological response of paediatric bone sarcomas using FDG PET in comparison to morphological volume measurement and standardized MRI parameters. Eur J Nucl Med Mol Imaging 2010;37: 1842–53.

57. Chang KJ, Kong CB, Cho WH, et al. Usefulness of increased 18F-FDG uptake for detecting local recurrence in patients with extremity osteosarcoma treated with surgical resection and endoprosthetic replacement. Skeletal Radiol 2015; 44(4):529–37.

58. Gupta K, Pawaskar A, Basu S, et al. Potential role of FDG PET imaging in predicting metastatic potential and assessment of therapeutic response to neoadjuvant chemotherapy in Ewing sarcoma family of tumors. Clin Nucl Med 2011;36(11): 973–7.

59. Treglia G, Salsano M, Stefanelli A, et al. Diagnostic accuracy of 18F-FDG-PET and PET/CT in patients with Ewing sarcoma family tumors: a systematic review and a meta-analysis. Skeletal Radiol 2012;41: 249–56.

60. Györke T, Zajic T, Lange A, et al. Impact of FDG PET for staging of Ewing sarcomas and primitive

neuroectodermal tumors. Nucl Med Commun 2006; 27:17–24.

61. Franzius C, Daldrup-Link HE, Wagner-Bohn A, et al. FDG-PET for detection of recurrences from malignant primary bone tumors: comparison with conventional imaging. Ann Oncol 2002;13:157–60.

62. Hawkins DS, Schuetze SM, Butrynski JE, et al. [18F] Fluorodeoxyglucose positron emission tomography predicts outcome for Ewing sarcoma family of tumors. J Clin Oncol 2005;23:8828–34.

63. Palmerini E, Colangeli M, Nanni C, et al. The role of FDG PET/CT in patients treated with neoadjuvant chemotherapy for localized bone sarcomas. Eur J Nucl Med Mol Imaging 2017;44(2):215–23.

64. Arush MW, Israel O, Postovsky S, et al. Positron emission tomography/computed tomography with 18fluoro-deoxyglucose in the detection of local recurrence and distant metastases of pediatric sarcoma. Pediatr Blood Cancer 2007;49(7):901–5.

65. Lee FY, Yu J, Chang SS, et al. Diagnostic value and limitations of fluorine-18 fluorodeoxyglucose positron emission tomography for cartilaginous tumors of bone. J Bone Joint Surg Am 2004;86-A:2677.

66. Jesus-Garcia R, Osawa A, Filippi RZ, et al. Is PET–CT an accurate method for the differential diagnosis between chondroma and chondrosarcoma? Springerplus 2016;5:236.

67. Purandare NC, Rangarajan V, Agarwal M, et al. Integrated PET/CT in evaluating sarcomatous transformation in osteochondromas. Clin Nucl Med 2009;34(6):350–4.

68. Brenner W, Conrad EU, Eary JF. FDG PET imaging for grading and prediction of outcome in chondrosarcoma patients. Eur J Nucl Med Mol Imaging 2004;31:189.

69. Osgood CL, Tantawy MN, Maloney N, et al. 18F-FLT positron emission tomography (PET) is a pharmacodynamic marker for EWS-FLI1 activity and Ewing sarcoma. Sci Rep 2016;6:33926.

70. Cobben DC, Elsinga PH, Suurmeijer AJ, et al. Detection and grading of soft tissue sarcomas of the extremities with (18)F-3'-fluoro-3'-deoxy-L-thymidine. Clin Cancer Res 2004;10:1685–90.

71. Benz MR, Czernin J, Allen-Auerbach MS, et al. 3'-deoxy-3'-[18F]fluorothymidine positron emission tomography for response assessment in soft tissue sarcoma: a pilot study to correlate imaging findings with tissue thymidine kinase 1 and Ki-67 activity and histopathologic response. Cancer 2012;118: 3135–44.

The Role of PET/MR Imaging in Precision Medicine

Eugene Huo, MD[a], David M. Wilson, MD[a],
Laura Eisenmenger, MD[a], Thomas A. Hope, MD[a,b],*

KEYWORDS

- PET/CT • PET/MR imaging • Precision medicine • Molecular imaging

KEY POINTS

- The superior capabilities of MR imaging to characterize soft tissue offers an advantage compared with computed tomography in the diagnosis of malignancy.
- PET tracers targeting specific pathologic processes can be more accurate and sensitive for primary and metastatic disease when compared with conventional contrast agents and nontargeted radiotracers.
- Precision PET tracers combined with MR imaging can provide diagnostic options unavailable with any other modality.
- PET tracers can be combined with radioactive sources to act as not just diagnostic agents but also radiotherapeutics.

INTRODUCTION

PET/computed tomography (CT) has become commonplace in the diagnosis and evaluation of malignancy; however, PET/MR imaging is emerging as a strong competitor with current and potential applications in precision medicine. Precision medicine is loosely defined as an approach to disease treatment and prevention that takes into account individual variability in the patient's tumor. As therapies have become more disease specific, diagnostic imaging must continue to advance with tailored disease-specific agents.

PET imaging has always provided valuable functional information about physiologic processes beyond simple evaluation of anatomy or lesion size. Using various combinations of radioisotopes and tracers, PET has advanced past identification of glucose metabolism and can now precisely identify specific disease processes, clusters of malignant cells, or mutations.[1] Through the development of new targeted molecular imaging methods, PET is better able to assay in vivo biological processes noninvasively and quantitatively, with the potential to identify patients with specific tumors or genotypes of disease.

Early studies have shown combining the use of these targeted precision medicine PET agents with MR imaging has some definite advantages compared with PET/CT. Unlike the low intrinsic soft tissue contrast of CT,[2] the superior soft tissue contrast of MR imaging allows for the improved assessment of fine anatomic detail[3–5] and can provide additional information on tissue composition and function not possible with CT. In allowing for more precise evaluation of disease-specific

Disclosure Statement: T.A. Hope receives research support from GE Healthcare.
[a] Department of Radiology and Biomedical Imaging, University of California San Francisco, 505 Parnassus Avenue, San Francisco, CA 94143, USA; [b] Department of Radiology, San Francisco VA Health Care System, 4150 Clement Street, San Francisco, CA 94121, USA
* Corresponding author. 505 Parnassus Avenue, M-391, San Francisco, CA 94143.
E-mail address: thomas.hope@ucsf.edu

PET Clin 12 (2017) 489–501
http://dx.doi.org/10.1016/j.cpet.2017.05.006
1556-8598/17/Published by Elsevier Inc.

markers in combination with excellent anatomic detail, PET/MR imaging offers a way not only to identify those patients who may benefit from targeted treatment but also a better method of evaluating disease response. This article reviews both the current and future directions of PET/MR imaging in precision medicine.

PET/MR IMAGING VERSUS PET/COMPUTED TOMOGRAPHY

PET/MR imaging as a modality is still in its fledgling stages but has shown much promise, with the unique information that can be obtained from both modalities. The current literature has begun to show that PET and MR imaging can be complementary in evaluating primary tumor, as well as assessing metastatic or recurrent disease.[6,7] There are 2 primary advantages of PET/MR imaging compared with PET/CT. First, with the advent of hybrid PET/MR imaging scanners that acquire and fuse metabolic information from PET with anatomic and functional data from MR imaging, it is now possible for complete spatial and temporal matching of PET and MR imaging data.[3,8] This is advantageous compared with the sequential nature of data acquisition inherent to PET/CT, reducing misregistration and allowing for easier transition of PET/MR imaging into the clinical setting.

The second major advantage is the superior soft tissue information provided by MR imaging. PET/CT may detect small foci of radionuclide uptake; however, due to the low soft tissue contrast of CT and the sequential data acquisition of PET/CT, lesion localization may suffer in some circumstances and anatomic correlates for small PET findings may be overlooked. The superior soft tissue contrast of MR imaging allows for the improved assessment of fine anatomic detail, including clear depiction of lesion margins, local tumor infiltration, and the relationship of lesions to adjacent structures.[3–5] MR imaging contrast agents can also provide specific imaging information regarding soft tissues, such as macrophage infiltration with the use of ferumoxytol and hepatobiliary imaging with gadoxetate disodium. With this fine anatomic detail and specialized contrast agents, PET/MR imaging will often help in detection of small lesions that may be difficult for either modality to demonstrate alone.

In addition to the anatomic detail and contrast enhancement, MR imaging is capable of providing functional information with diffusion-weighted imaging (DWI), perfusion imaging, and spectroscopy not possible with CT and without the use of ionizing radiation. DWI has proven particularly valuable in the assessment of lesion cellularity,

and may be used as a whole-body screening technique for the detection of neoplastic lesions, including small lesions less than 10 mm in diameter.[9,10] Magnetic resonance spectroscopy's ability to detect metabolites can also help to differentiate normal versus abnormal tissue and distinguish proliferation versus necrosis in masses.[11] Dynamic contrast-enhanced MR imaging can be used to evaluate lesion perfusion, with certain malignant lesions demonstrating characteristic perfusion patterns.[12] This functional information can further assist in diagnosis and evaluation of disease response.

Even though there are many potential advantages, PET/MR imaging does have some disadvantages. Because MR imaging cannot directly measure density, alternative methods of attenuation-correction must be used.[13] The cost of a combined PET/MR imaging scanner is greater than the combined cost of a separate PET and MR imaging scanner, while decreasing the flexibility in utilization. Specific body regions are known to have decreased imaging sensitivity on PET/MR imaging compared with PET/CT, including evaluation of bowel-based tumors due to peristaltic motion and in the evaluation for pulmonary nodules.[14] Despite these limitations, the combination of PET and MR imaging has already proven to be helpful with the use of ^{18}F-fluorodeoxyglucose (FDG), and may have increased utility when applied to precision medicine.

Issues related to attenuation correction with PET/MR imaging cannot be overlooked when considering precision medicine. Accurate quantification of uptake is critical for tumor characterization and inclusion of imaging modalities in clinical trials. Quantitative accuracy in PET relies on 2 main processes: attenuation correction and PET reconstruction parameters. In PET/CT, measurement of attenuation maps is straightforward because the CT component measures density directly. Therefore, phantoms used in PET/CT disregard attenuation as a source of error and methods to evaluate quantitative accuracy focus on PET reconstruction parameters. Using PET/CT phantoms, one can create protocols that deliver reproducible PET quantification.[15,16] These same phantoms cannot be used in PET/MR imaging because the phantoms cannot reproduce the MR imaging and density characteristics that would be required to evaluate the accuracy of the attenuation map produced in PET/MR imaging. Additionally, these phantoms create significant artifacts when imaged using MR imaging due to the materials they are made of.[17,18] Currently, when one measures activity in a phantom in PET/MR imaging, a predetermined density map is used for attenuation rather than one acquired directly from the phantom at the time of imaging. In particular, this is relevant for the pelvis, where bone is not included in the attenuation map in the currently commercially available systems, which can result in a 20% error in quantitative accuracy.[19,20] It is imperative that radiologists develop phantoms and reconstruction parameters specific to PET/MR imaging to delineate the quantitative error in PET/MR imaging. This will allow PET/MR imaging to be included in multicenter clinical trials and verify that the measured uptake is accurate and valid, thereby making it appropriate for use in precision medicine applications.

PRECISION MEDICINE

Many malignancies in the past have been treated by surgery, radiation, or generalized chemotherapies, but more and more frequently treatments are more targeted.[21–24] Although not all patients respond to targeted therapies, those patients who harbor specific mutations can be given therapy directed specifically to the tumor genotype. The tumor molecular profile can also be used to predict prognosis and response to therapy.[1] Some of these some principles can and are being applied to PET/MR imaging.

PET imaging can take 2 major forms: nontargeted imaging and targeted molecular imaging. Nontargeted molecular imaging typically images cellular processes, such as glucose metabolism and cell proliferation. Because this method focuses on general cellular processes, it often does not characterize individual patient's tumors. For targeted molecular imaging, probes directly image specific molecular targets, such as transporters or enzymes. Both nontargeted molecular imaging and targeted molecular imaging can be useful in disease diagnosis and monitoring (see later discussion).

POTENTIAL OF HYPERPOLARIZED MR IMAGING

One aspect of MR imaging that has not yet been used in the setting of PET/MR imaging is hyperpolarized MR imaging. New MR imaging–compatible molecular imaging techniques have the potential to identify cancer and other diseases, providing metabolic information that has traditionally been the domain of high-sensitivity methods like PET.[25,26] Specifically, hyperpolarized ^{13}C MR imaging uses a recently developed technique, solution dynamic nuclear polarization (DNP), to dramatically increase the signal of ^{13}C-enriched metabolic agents. The resulting increase in sensitivity (up to 10^6) allows real-time observation of metabolism in living systems, based on the conversion of an introduced ^{13}C substrate into its metabolic products. Metabolism is observed by new resonances in the hyperpolarized ^{13}C spectrum, reflecting the subtle frequency shift between different ^{13}C small molecules in vivo.

One important target has been pyruvate, a 3-carbon molecule that sits at the crossroads of human metabolism. In cancer, pyruvate is converted primarily to lactate, reflecting the glycolytic phenotype observed in many human neoplasms. This conversion can typically be observed within the first few seconds of introducing hyperpolarized ^{13}C pyruvate into human cancers, including those of the prostate, brain, and liver.[27] Although hyperpolarized ^{13}C MR imaging is a relatively new technology (solution DNP was first reported in 2003), a wealth of data has been generated in cell and animal models relevant to human cancer.[28] Furthermore, the method is not limited to ^{13}C pyruvate, with numerous newer probes applied to study in vivo perfusion, reduction and oxidation (redox), pH, necrosis, and glutaminolysis.

A successful in vivo hyperpolarized ^{13}C MR imaging experiment requires expertise in chemistry, biochemistry, engineering, pulse sequence design, pharmaceutical sciences, and data processing. Not surprisingly, successful use in humans has been challenging, with the potential of the method recently met in a first-in-human clinical trial in subjects with prostate cancer.[29] This study demonstrated the safety of ^{13}C pyruvate in a series of subjects with cancer, and showed that both hyperpolarized ^{13}C pyruvate and its metabolic product ^{13}C lactate could be detected in the human prostate. Future work will extend this method to other human cancers, including those of the brain (glioblastoma multiforme) and liver (metastatic breast cancer). To extend this technology into widespread clinical practice, there are ongoing efforts to improve coil design and data acquisition, as well as to engineer robust solution DNP systems. Furthermore, combined modality imaging such as PET/MR imaging highlights the potential of using multiple metabolic techniques in tandem to better diagnose and treat the metabolic disturbances in patients with cancer. PET is typically limited to 1 targeted probe; however, the combination of hyperpolarized MR imaging and PET allows for the simultaneous imaging of multiple targets and pathways.

NONTARGETED MOLECULAR PROBES

Currently, PET/MR imaging is primarily used with less specific nontargeted molecular imaging agents. Through the imaging of cell processes, nontargeted molecular imaging can be used to identify abnormal cell physiology and monitor cellular changes over time. Nontargeted molecular probes are radiolabeled versions of compounds used or retained in higher amounts within a targeted pathologic process when compared with normal physiologic ones. The most common cellular processes imaged by nontargeted molecular imaging and PET/MR imaging are glucose metabolism (^{18}F-FDG), lipogenesis (^{11}C-choline, ^{11}C-acetate), cellular proliferation or DNA synthesis (^{18}F-fluorothymidine, ^{18}F-FMAU), and cellular hypoxia (^{18}F-fluoromisonidazole, nitroimidazole compounds).

The most commonly used nontargeted agent is FDG PET (**Fig. 1**). Because glucose metabolism is not specific to tumors, areas of naturally high or increased metabolism also demonstrate increased uptake, such as the brain, heart, or bowel, in addition to inflammatory or infectious processes. Despite the limitations of ^{18}FDG, the information from a PET scan when combined with the soft-tissue resolution of MR imaging has resulted in an examination that can affect treatment decisions. Rectal cancer is among the

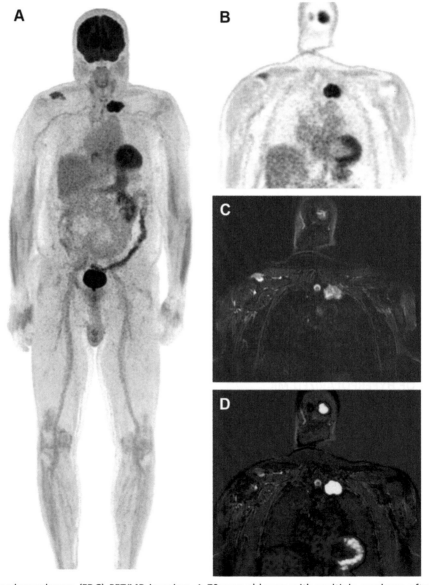

Fig. 1. Fluorodeoxyglucose (FDG) PET/MR imaging. A 79-year-old man with multiple myeloma after radiation, stem cell transplant, and thalidomide. (*A*) MIP and (*B*) coronal PET images demonstrations uptake within the left lung apex and right shoulder, corresponding to active disease. Corresponding (*C*) short tau inversion recovery and (*D*) fused PET/MR imaging images.

diseases that have the potential to benefit from the combination of modalities.

Treatment of rectal cancer changes greatly based on both the presence of distant metastatic disease and local T-staging. MR imaging is the best current imaging modality for identifying depth of invasion, which is the key prognostic factor in determining T-stage. Preoperative radiation therapy has a high morbidity when given in T1, T2, and early T3 disease but offers a reduction in recurrence rate postresection when given in advanced T3 or greater disease. However, detection of nodal and metastatic disease is extremely variable, depending on the reader, and requires a significant amount of expertise.[30] Metastatic disease is most commonly found in the liver and lymph nodes, and although distant disease changes the treatment algorithm, resection is still possible. PET has been shown to significantly improve the detection of disease compared with CT alone, revealing unknown disease in 19% of patients, and changing the therapeutic approach 17% of patients.[31] PET also has a role in the evaluation of rectal cancer after resection,

successfully differentiating recurrent or residual rectal cancer from scar.[32]

[18]F-choline is a nontargeted molecular probe that demonstrates increased uptake in prostate and parathyroid cancers due to increased choline kinase activity and increased choline transport.[33,34] PET/MR imaging with ^{18}F-choline has been shown to improve the detection rate of prostate cancer in targeted biopsies compared with MR imaging alone.[35] ^{18}F-choline agents have shown better detection of both androgen-dependent and independent prostate cancers in vitro.[36] A few studies have noted the discovery of incidental parathyroid adenomas on[18]F-choline PET/MR imaging studies for prostate cancer staging[37–39] (**Fig. 2**). One pilot study demonstrated an 89% sensitivity and 100% specificity for identification of histologically confirmed adenomas in patients with prior inconclusive ultrasound and [99]mTc-sestamibi scintigraphy. PET/MR imaging not only located the responsible adenomas but also was able to provide detailed anatomic information to the surgeons.[40] Because the sensitivity of conventional dual-tracer subtraction scintigraphy using

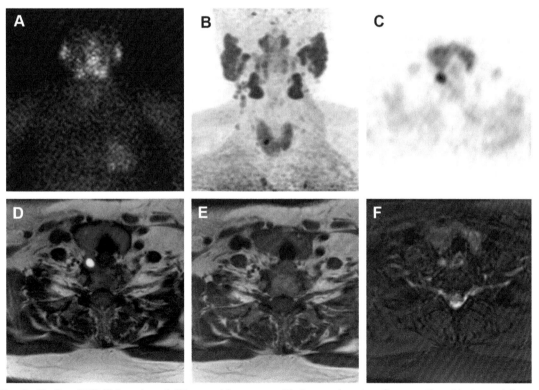

Fig. 2. Choline PET/MR imaging. A 65-year-old woman with hypercalcemia, after parathyroidectomy. Isthmus nodule detected on ultrasound with a benign biopsy and (*A*) negative sestamibi scan. A focus of uptake on choline PET/MR imaging (*B*) MIP and (*C*) axial images was identified posterior to the right thyroid lobe. (*D*) Fused PET/MR imaging images demonstrate the right paraesophageal adenoma with (*E*) T1 hypointensity and (*F*) T2 hyperintensity.

^{99}mTc-tetrofosmin and ^{123}I coupled with ultrasonography drops to as low as 30% if multiple parathyroid glands are involved,[41–44] dynamic contrast-enhanced CT and ^{18}F-choline PET/CT have emerged as imaging modalities that can identify these subtle parathyroid adenomas.[37,45–49]

TARGETED MOLECULAR IMAGING

Targeted molecular imaging images specific molecular targets such as transporters or enzymes, which have the potential to be earlier and more sensitive biomarkers of therapeutic efficacy. In addition, many preclinical and clinical studies suggest that targeted molecular imaging provides useful methods for monitoring targeted therapy in PET/MR imaging. The targeted molecular imaging probes in common use can be divided by different targeted ligands, monoclonal antibodies or their fragments, natural peptide ligands or their analogues, tyrosine kinase inhibitors or their analogues, and high-affinity peptides. Precision medicine PET/MR imaging with targeted molecular imaging is being applied in a few disease processes currently, most commonly in prostate and neuroendocrine tumor (NET).

Prostate Carcinoma

For the evaluation of prostate cancer, MR imaging is known to be superior to CT,[50] gaining acceptance in American Urological Association guidelines.[51] CT has not been shown to have a role in prostate cancer evaluation except for the identification of nodal disease and evaluation of sclerotic osseous metastases.[50] For evaluation of the primary tumor, multiparametric MR imaging (mpMR imaging) combines anatomic and functional MR imaging, including T2-weighted, DWI, and dynamic-contrast enhanced MR imaging.[52] The diffusion component of mpMR imaging is the strongest predictive factor of cancer in the peripheral zone,[53] which is reflected in the weight given to it in the Prostate Imaging Reporting and Data System (PIRADS) version 2 reporting system.[52] Newer studies have shown that DWI can also predict tumor grading[54,55] in the peripheral zone and may have a role as a predictive biomarker for biochemical recurrence.[56]

There have been several new developments over the past 5 years in the imaging of prostate cancer, including probes-targeting bombesin[57] and prostate-specific membrane antigen (PSMA). PMSA is a transmembrane protein expressed in high levels in more than 90% of prostate carcinomas.[58] The expression of PMSA correlates with unfavorable prognostic factors, such as a high Gleason score, infiltrative growth, metastasis, and hormone independence.[58] 68-gallium (^{68}Ga)-PSMA has demonstrated a high sensitivity and specificity for prostate cancer, allowing for detection of even small amounts of tumor, both local and metastatic.[59–61] The most commonly used PSMA-targeted probe is ^{68}Ga-PSMA N,N'-bis [2-hydroxy-5-(carboxyethyl)benzyl] ethylenediamine-N,N'-diacetic acid (HBED-CC or PSMA-11).[62]

The 4 main applications of imaging in prostate cancer are in patients with low-risk disease, evaluation of high-risk preprostatectomy patients, post-treatment biochemical recurrence, and CRPC.

Active surveillance describes the observation of patients with lower grade biopsies (Gleason score <6) who may not benefit from definitive therapy. In this approach, immediate radical prostatectomy or radiation therapy is deferred in favor of continuous surveillance.[63] To date, there has been no evaluation of patients under active surveillance, although there is the belief that the combination of MR imaging and PET could detect clinically significant cancers. Currently, there is a clinical trial evaluating a PSMA targeted compound in active surveillance patients but without MR imaging for comparison (NCT02615067).[64] This is a large unmet need and the combination of hyperpolarized MR imaging with PET may have better imaging characteristics than MR imaging alone.[27] Eiber and colleagues[65] compared PET/MR imaging with the already established mpMR imaging, as well as the PET, and found that ^{68}Ga-PSMA-11 PET/MR imaging had a higher diagnostic accuracy than either mpMR imaging or PET alone for the evaluation of the primary tumor (**Fig. 3**). This study was in subjects with intermediate to high-grade tumors in which detection of the primary tumor is not as critical; however, it does suggest that this approach may be applicable in the active surveillance population.

The most common classification schema for risk stratification of patients with prostate cancer is the D'Amico criteria.[66] Approximately 15% of patients diagnosed with prostate cancer fit into this category. With a diagnosis of high-risk prostate cancer, 22% have osseous metastases and 33% have pelvic nodal disease.[67] With the high specificities in detecting nodal and osseous metastatic disease, PET/MR imaging can be useful in the evaluation of these patients before definitive therapy. Initial studies have been performed evaluating PSMA PET for nodal staging of high-risk patients[68] but comparisons between PET/CT and PET/MR imaging have not yet been performed.

Biochemical recurrence is defined as an elevation in prostate-specific antigen (PSA) of greater than 0.2 ng/mL after treatment, confirmed by a second

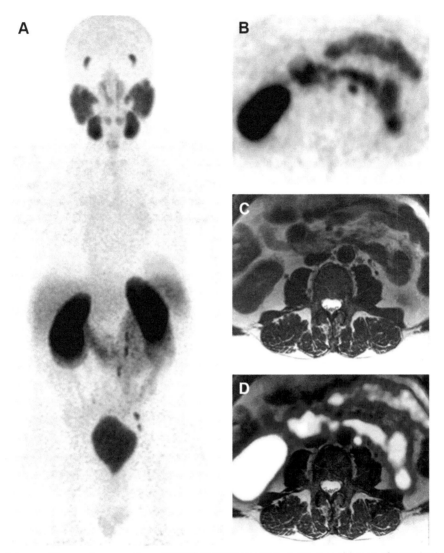

Fig. 3. Prostate-specific membrane antigen (PSMA) PET/MR imaging. A 67-year-old man after radical prostatectomy and external beam radiation treatment, now with biochemical recurrence, prostate-specific antigen = 6.1. (A) PSMA maximum intensity projection (MIP) and (B) axial images demonstrate uptake in multiple retroperitoneal lymph nodes also seen on T2 MR imaging (C) but are more readily identified on (D) fused PET/MR imaging images. Based on the imaging findings, management was changed from planned pelvic salvage radiation to monotherapy with androgen deprivation therapy.

test.[69] Up to 32% of patients after radical-prostatectomy and 41% of patients postradiation therapy will have recurrence.[70,71] Afshar-Oromieh and colleagues[72] used ^{68}Ga-PSMA-11 to demonstrate the superiority of PET/MR imaging to PET/CT in prostate cancer evaluation. This study noted that the higher lesion contrast and higher imaging resolution of MR imaging enabled a subjectively easier evaluation, in addition to classifying unclear findings on PET/CT as characteristic of prostate cancer metastases on PET/MR imaging. Freitag and colleagues[73] also demonstrated the additional value of using mpMR imaging in a PET/MR imaging

protocol. In this study, the ^{68}Ga-PSMA-11 PET-component of either PET/MR imaging or PET/CT found at least 1 pathologic lesion in 93 out of 119 subjects with an additional 18 out of 119 subjects (15.1%) diagnosed with a local recurrence in multiparametric portion of the PET/MR imaging. This demonstrated the additional value of hybrid ^{68}Ga-PSMA-11 PET/MR imaging by gaining complementary diagnostic information from mpMR imaging compared with the capabilities of PET/CT.

Castrate-resistant prostate cancer (CRPC) describes patients with persistent elevation of their

PSA despite a low level of testosterone, typically while being treated with androgen-deprivation therapy. CRPC still responds to secondary hormonal treatments that target the androgen receptor. CRPC also demonstrates increased PSMA expression,[74] which enables PSMA-labeled radiopharmaceuticals to be used for imaging and therapy of CRPC. Early attempts with PSMA-directed radiolabeled ligands with antibodies were limited by the slow clearance and toxicity.[40] PSMA radioligand therapy with ^{177}Lu-PSMA showed at least a partial response in 56% of subjects,[75] with less overall toxicity than the PSMA antibody treatments [177]LU-DOTA (1,4,7,10-tetraazacyclododecane-1,4,7,10-tetraacetic acid)-J591.[76] Median progression-free survival was at least comparable to other treatments for CRPC. Although the role of PSMA peptide receptor radionuclide therapy (PRRT) has yet to be determined, PET/MR imaging may play a role for patient selection and evaluation of disease response in these patients.

NEUROENDOCRINE TUMORS

Another area that has been under investigation for the utility of precision medicine in PET/MR imaging is NETs. NETs include a variety of tumor types; however, well-differentiated NETs express somatostatin receptors (SSTRs), particularly type 2 receptors.[77] NETs are generally slow-growing and clinically indolent. Accurate localization and evaluation of the full extent of NET disease burden is important to determine treatment options. Up to 13% of patients present with metastatic disease, and 75% of small bowel NET and up to 85% of pancreatic NET patients are discovered to have hepatic metastatic disease during the course of their disease.[78] In many of these patients, detection and possibly treatment with PRRT may offer their only chance in changing the course of disease.[79]

In the last 15 years, ^{68}Ga-labeled peptides targeting SSTRs have been developed, demonstrating increased sensitivity compared with octreotide for the evaluation of NETs.[80,81] These

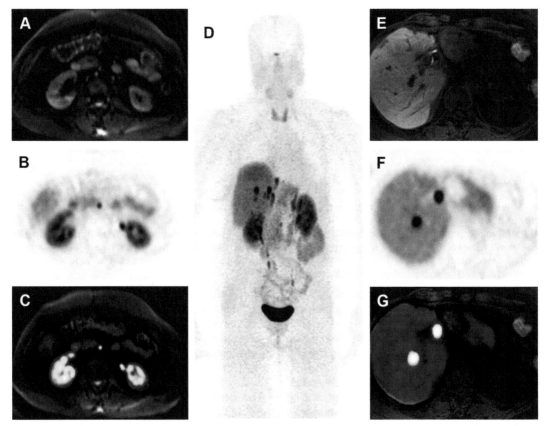

Fig. 4. DOTA-TOC PET/MR imaging. A 71-year-old woman with pancreatic neuroendocrine tumor after left hepatectomy and pancreatectomy. Multiple hepatic metastatic lesions previously treated with bland embolization. Retroperitoneal lymph nodes are noted on (A) diffusion-weighted imaging (DWI) b = 600 imaging but only 1 has increased (B, C) DOTA-TOC uptake. PET (D) MIP also demonstrates multiple hepatic imaging seen on axial (E) hepatobiliary phase, (F) PET, and (G) fusion images.

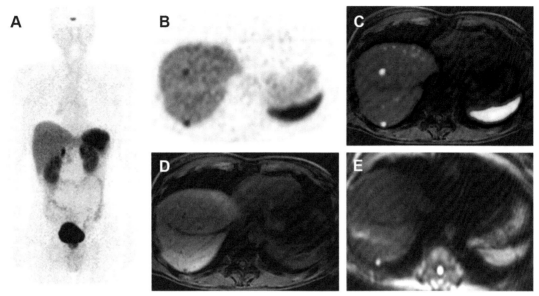

Fig. 5. DOTA (1,4,7,10-tetraazacyclododecane-1,4,7,10-tetraacetic acid)-D-Phe1-Tyr3-octreotide (TOC) PET/MR imaging. Small bowel NET status after partial hepatectomy for metastatic disease. PET (A) MIP, (B) axial, and (C) fused PET/MR imaging images demonstrate 2 small lesions with DOTA-TOC uptake. On (D) hepatobiliary phase and (E) diffusion-weighted imaging, only the posterior lesion is visible.

agents include DOTA-D-Phe1-Tyr3-octreotide (DOTA-TOC), DOTA-1-Nal3-octreotide (DOTA-NOC), and DOTA-DPhe1-Tyr3-octreotate (DOTA-TATE).[80,81] In addition to the improvement in sensitivity and spatial resolution, ^{68}Ga-labeled peptides can be used in both PET/CT and PET/MR imaging and also provide patients with shorter examinations and less radiation exposure than Octreoscan examinations.[82]

Gaertner and colleagues[83] conducted one of the first studies to demonstrate that anatomic correlates to ^{68}Ga-DOTA-TOC PET were significantly better delineated on MR imaging compared with CT images, and that there was better coregistration of functional and morphologic data on PET/MR imaging. This study proved at least equivalence of ^{68}Ga-DOTA-TOC PET/MR imaging and PET/CT. Other early investigations have suggested that PET/MR imaging has some advantages compared with PET/CT that can improve detection of NET metastatic disease.[84] MR imaging has higher sensitivity for hepatic lesion detection compared with CT due to DWI and the hepatobiliary agent gadoxetate disodium (Eovist, Bayer Healthcare, Wayne, NJ, USA)[85–88] (**Figs. 4** and **5**). For example, hepatobiliary phase MR imaging detected 99% of hepatic metastasis compared with 46% for CT and 64% for PET (P<.001).[84,89] Additionally, the anatomic detail provided by the MR imaging component of PET/MR imaging is useful in compensating for the decreased uptake in poorly differentiated NETs from decreased SSTR expression.[90]

Targeted agents selective for SSTRs have also been developed for therapeutic uses. Tumors with high expression of SSTRs detected by diagnostic imaging agents are also excellent targets for PRRT. ^{90}Y-DOTA-TOC and ^{177}Lu-DOTA-TATE have been used for therapy, especially useful in patients who have failed treatments with first-line somatostatin analogues. A recently concluded trial compared 229 subjects with metastatic midgut NETs treated with ^{177}Lu-DOTA-TATE or high-dose octreotide-long-acting release; there was a 79% lower risk of progression or death in the ^{177}Lu-DOTA-TATE group.[79] The role of imaging for patient selection and treatment response has yet to be determined but, given that less than 20% of subjects demonstrated a radiographic response in the trial, PET/MR imaging may play a role in determining how patients have responded to therapy.

SUMMARY

With the development of more targeted therapies for the treatment of malignancy, earlier and more accurate identification of treatment response could prove essential in improving patient outcomes. Although clinical studies have suggested that targeted molecular imaging can provide a useful method for monitoring targeted therapy in PET/MR imaging, there are currently several barriers limiting the research and clinical use of PET/MR imaging precision medicine.

Major barriers include the relatively small numbers of PET agents approved by the US Food and Drug Administration, accessibility to PET/MR imaging scanners, and relative lack of data supporting the use of PET/MR imaging compared with PET/CT using these tracers. Despite this, progress is being made in demonstrating the superiority of PET/MR imaging compared with PET/CT, including applications in targeted evaluation of prostate cancer, NETs, and parathyroid disease. It is hoped that these studies and larger clinical trials will lay the groundwork for determining clinical indications and standardizing PET/MR imaging protocols. With current and continued development in both PET and MR technology, PET/MR imaging will be a large contributor in precision medicine now and in the future.

REFERENCES

1. Teng FF, Meng X, Sun XD, et al. New strategy for monitoring targeted therapy: molecular imaging. Int J Nanomedicine 2013;8:3703–13.
2. Catalano OA, Masch WR, Catana C, et al. An overview of PET/MR, focused on clinical applications. Abdom Radiol (NY) 2017;42(2):631–44.
3. Delso G, Furst S, Jakoby B, et al. Performance measurements of the Siemens mMR integrated whole-body PET/MR scanner. J Nucl Med 2011;52(12):1914–22.
4. Torigian DA, Zaidi H, Kwee TC, et al. PET/MR imaging: technical aspects and potential clinical applications. Radiology 2013;267(1):26–44.
5. von Schulthess GK, Schlemmer HP. A look ahead: PET/MR versus PET/CT. Eur J Nucl Med Mol Imaging 2009;36(Suppl 1):S3–9.
6. Drzezga A, Souvatzoglou M, Eiber M, et al. First clinical experience with integrated whole-body PET/MR: comparison to PET/CT in patients with oncologic diagnoses. J Nucl Med 2012;53(6):845–55.
7. Al-Nabhani KZ, Syed R, Michopoulou S, et al. Qualitative and quantitative comparison of PET/CT and PET/MR imaging in clinical practice. J Nucl Med 2014;55(1):88–94.
8. Zaidi H, Ojha N, Morich M, et al. Design and performance evaluation of a whole-body Ingenuity TF PET-MRI system. Phys Med Biol 2011;56(10):3091–106.
9. Nasu K, Kuroki Y, Nawano S, et al. Hepatic metastases: diffusion-weighted sensitivity-encoding versus SPIO-enhanced MR imaging. Radiology 2006;239(1):122–30.
10. Padhani AR, Koh DM, Collins DJ. Whole-body diffusion-weighted MR imaging in cancer: current status and research directions. Radiology 2011;261(3):700–18.
11. Nguyen ML, Willows B, Khan R, et al. The potential role of magnetic resonance spectroscopy in image-guided radiotherapy. Front Oncol 2014;4:91.
12. Fusco R, Sansone M, Filice S, et al. Pattern recognition approaches for breast cancer DCE-MRI classification: a systematic review. J Med Biol Eng 2016;36(4):449–59.
13. Delso G, ter Voert E, de Galiza Barbosa F, et al. Pitfalls and limitations in simultaneous PET/MRI. Semin Nucl Med 2015;45(6):552–9.
14. Chandarana H, Heacock L, Rakheja R, et al. Pulmonary nodules in patients with primary malignancy: comparison of hybrid PET/MR and PET/CT imaging. Radiology 2013;268(3):874–81.
15. Sunderland JJ, Christian PE. Quantitative PET/CT scanner performance characterization based upon the society of nuclear medicine and molecular imaging clinical trials network oncology clinical simulator phantom. J Nucl Med 2015;56(1):145–52.
16. Fahey FH, Kinahan PE, Doot RK, et al. Variability in PET quantitation within a multicenter consortium. Med Phys 2010;37(7):3660–6.
17. Tropp J. Image brightening in samples of high dielectric constant. J Magn Reson 2004;167(1):12–24.
18. Ziegler S, Braun H, Ritt P, et al. Systematic evaluation of phantom fluids for simultaneous PET/MR hybrid imaging. J Nucl Med 2013;54(8):1464–71.
19. Samarin A, Burger C, Wollenweber SD, et al. PET/MR imaging of bone lesions–implications for PET quantification from imperfect attenuation correction. Eur J Nucl Med Mol Imaging 2012;39(7):1154–60.
20. Leynes AP, Yang J, Shanbhag DD, et al. Hybrid ZTE/Dixon MR-based attenuation correction for quantitative uptake estimation of pelvic lesions in PET/MRI. Med Phys 2017;44(3):902–13.
21. Ou SH. Crizotinib: a novel and first-in-class multitargeted tyrosine kinase inhibitor for the treatment of anaplastic lymphoma kinase rearranged non-small cell lung cancer and beyond. Drug Des Devel Ther 2011;5:471–85.
22. Moon YW, Park S, Sohn JH, et al. Clinical significance of progesterone receptor and HER2 status in estrogen receptor-positive, operable breast cancer with adjuvant tamoxifen. J Cancer Res Clin Oncol 2011;137(7):1123–30.
23. Scartozzi M, Bearzi I, Berardi R, et al. Epidermal growth factor receptor (EGFR) status in primary colorectal tumors does not correlate with EGFR expression in related metastatic sites: implications for treatment with EGFR-targeted monoclonal antibodies. J Clin Oncol 2004;22(23):4772–8.
24. Zidan J, Dashkovsky I, Stayerman C, et al. Comparison of HER-2 overexpression in primary breast cancer and metastatic sites and its effect on biological

targeting therapy of metastatic disease. Br J Cancer 2005;93(5):552–6.

25. Di Gialleonardo V, Wilson DM, Keshari KR. The potential of metabolic imaging. Semin Nucl Med 2016;46(1):28–39.

26. Kurhanewicz J, Bok R, Nelson SJ, et al. Current and potential applications of clinical 13C MR spectroscopy. J Nucl Med 2008;49(3):341–4.

27. Wilson DM, Kurhanewicz J. Hyperpolarized 13C MR for molecular imaging of prostate cancer. J Nucl Med 2014;55(10):1567–72.

28. Keshari KR, Wilson DM. Chemistry and biochemistry of 13C hyperpolarized magnetic resonance using dynamic nuclear polarization. Chem Soc Rev 2014; 43(5):1627–59.

29. Nelson SJ, Kurhanewicz J, Vigneron DB, et al. Metabolic imaging of patients with prostate cancer using hyperpolarized [1-(1)(3)C]pyruvate. Sci Transl Med 2013;5(198):198ra108.

30. Kaur H, Choi H, You YN, et al. MR imaging for preoperative evaluation of primary rectal cancer: practical considerations. Radiographics 2012; 32(2):389–409.

31. Shin SS, Jeong YY, Min JJ, et al. Preoperative staging of colorectal cancer: CT vs. integrated FDG PET/CT. Abdom Imaging 2008;33(3):270–7.

32. Ito K, Kato T, Tadokoro M, et al. Recurrent rectal cancer and scar: differentiation with PET and MR imaging. Radiology 1992;182(2):549–52.

33. Ramirez de Molina A, Rodriguez-Gonzalez A, Gutierrez R, et al. Overexpression of choline kinase is a frequent feature in human tumor-derived cell lines and in lung, prostate, and colorectal human cancers. Biochem Biophys Res Commun 2002; 296(3):580–3.

34. Awwad HM, Geisel J, Obeid R. The role of choline in prostate cancer. Clin Biochem 2012;45(18):1548–53.

35. Piert M, Montgomery J, Kunju LP, et al. 18F-Choline PET/MRI: the additional value of PET for MRI-guided transrectal prostate biopsies. J Nucl Med 2016; 57(7):1065–70.

36. Price DT, Coleman RE, Liao RP, et al. Comparison of [18F]Fluorocholine and [18F]Fluorodeoxyglucose for positron emission tomography of androgen dependent and androgen independent prostate cancer. J Urol 2002;168(1):273–80.

37. Cazaentre T, Clivaz F, Triponez F. False-positive result in 18F-fluorocholine PET/CT due to incidental and ectopic parathyroid hyperplasia. Clin Nucl Med 2014;39(6):e328–30.

38. Mapelli P, Busnardo E, Magnani P, et al. Incidental finding of parathyroid adenoma with 11C-choline PET/CT. Clin Nucl Med 2012;37(6):593–5.

39. Hodolic M, Huchet V, Balogova S, et al. Incidental uptake of (18)F-fluorocholine (FCH) in the head or in the neck of patients with prostate cancer. Radiol Oncol 2014;48(3):228–34.

40. Bouchelouche K, Turkbey B, Choyke PL. PSMA PET and radionuclide therapy in prostate cancer. Semin Nucl Med 2016;46(6):522–35.

41. Borley NR, Collins RE, O'Doherty M, et al. Technetium-99m sestamibi parathyroid localization is accurate enough for scan-directed unilateral neck exploration. Br J Surg 1996;83(7):989–91.

42. Hindie E, Melliere D, Jeanguillaume C, et al. Unilateral surgery for primary hyperparathyroidism on the basis of technetium Tc 99m sestamibi and iodine 123 subtraction scanning. Arch Surg 2000;135(12): 1461–8.

43. Johnston LB, Carroll MJ, Britton KE, et al. The accuracy of parathyroid gland localization in primary hyperparathyroidism using sestamibi radionuclide imaging. J Clin Endocrinol Metab 1996;81(1): 346–52.

44. Rubello D, Pelizzo MR, Casara D. Nuclear medicine and minimally invasive surgery of parathyroid adenomas: a fair marriage. Eur J Nucl Med Mol Imaging 2003;30(2):189–92.

45. Hoang JK, Sung WK, Bahl M, et al. How to perform parathyroid 4D CT: tips and traps for technique and interpretation. Radiology 2014;270(1):15–24.

46. Bahl M, Muzaffar M, Vij G, et al. Prevalence of the polar vessel sign in parathyroid adenomas on the arterial phase of 4D CT. AJNR Am J Neuroradiol 2014;35(3):578–81.

47. Orevi M, Freedman N, Mishani E, et al. Localization of parathyroid adenoma by (1)(1)C-choline PET/CT: preliminary results. Clin Nucl Med 2014;39(12): 1033–8.

48. van Raalte DH, Vlot MC, Zwijnenburg A, et al. F18-Choline PET/CT: a novel tool to localize parathyroid adenoma? Clin Endocrinol (Oxf) 2015; 82(6):910–2.

49. Lezaic L, Rep S, Sever MJ, et al. (1)(8)F-Fluorocholine PET/CT for localization of hyperfunctioning parathyroid tissue in primary hyperparathyroidism: a pilot study. Eur J Nucl Med Mol Imaging 2014;41(11): 2083–9.

50. Hricak H, Choyke PL, Eberhardt SC, et al. Imaging prostate cancer: a multidisciplinary perspective. Radiology 2007;243(1):28–53.

51. Rosenkrantz AB, Verma S, Choyke P, et al. Prostate magnetic resonance imaging and magnetic resonance imaging targeted biopsy in patients with a prior negative biopsy: a consensus statement by AUA and SAR. J Urol 2016;196(6):1613–8.

52. Weinreb JC, Barentsz JO, Choyke PL, et al. PI-RADS prostate imaging - reporting and data system: 2015, version 2. Eur Urol 2016;69(1):16–40.

53. Westphalen AC, Rosenkrantz AB. Prostate imaging reporting and data system (PI-RADS): reflections on early experience with a standardized interpretation scheme for multiparametric prostate MRI. AJR Am J Roentgenol 2014;202(1):121–3.

54. NiMhurchu E, O'Kelly F, Murphy IG, et al. Predictive value of PI-RADS classification in MRI-directed transrectal ultrasound guided prostate biopsy. Clin Radiol 2016;71(4):375–80.

55. Kim TH, Kim CK, Park BK, et al. Relationship between Gleason score and apparent diffusion coefficients of diffusion-weighted magnetic resonance imaging in prostate cancer patients. Can Urol Assoc J 2016;10(11–12):E377–82.

56. Park SY, Kim CK, Park BK, et al. Prediction of biochemical recurrence following radical prostatectomy in men with prostate cancer by diffusion-weighted magnetic resonance imaging: initial results. Eur Radiol 2011;21(5):1111–8.

57. Mansi R, Minamimoto R, Macke H, et al. Bombesin-targeted PET of prostate cancer. J Nucl Med 2016; 57(Suppl 3):67s–72s.

58. Kratochwil C, Afshar-Oromieh A, Kopka K, et al. Current status of prostate-specific membrane antigen targeting in nuclear medicine: clinical translation of chelator containing prostate-specific membrane antigen ligands into diagnostics and therapy for prostate cancer. Semin Nucl Med 2016;46(5):405–18.

59. Eiber M, Maurer T, Souvatzoglou M, et al. Evaluation of Hybrid (6)(8)Ga-PSMA Ligand PET/CT in 248 patients with biochemical recurrence after radical prostatectomy. J Nucl Med 2015;56(5):668–74.

60. Perera M, Papa N, Christidis D, et al. Sensitivity, specificity, and predictors of positive 68Ga-Prostate-specific membrane antigen positron emission tomography in advanced prostate cancer: a systematic review and meta-analysis. Eur Urol 2016;70(6): 926–37.

61. Freitag MT, Radtke JP, Hadaschik BA, et al. Comparison of hybrid (68)Ga-PSMA PET/MRI and (68)Ga-PSMA PET/CT in the evaluation of lymph node and bone metastases of prostate cancer. Eur J Nucl Med Mol Imaging 2016;43(1):70–83.

62. Afshar-Oromieh A, Malcher A, Eder M, et al. PET imaging with a [68Ga]gallium-labelled PSMA ligand for the diagnosis of prostate cancer: biodistribution in humans and first evaluation of tumour lesions. Eur J Nucl Med Mol Imaging 2013;40(4):486–95.

63. Chen RC, Rumble RB, Loblaw DA, et al. Active surveillance for the management of localized prostate cancer (Cancer Care Ontario Guideline): American Society of Clinical Oncology Clinical Practice Guideline Endorsement. J Clin Oncol 2016;34(18): 2182–90.

64. Molecular Insight Pharmaceuticals I. Study to evaluate 99mTc-MIP-1404 SPECT/CT imaging in men with biopsy proven low-grade prostate cancer. 2015. Available at: https://ClinicalTrials.gov/show/NCT02615067.

65. Eiber M, Weirich G, Holzapfel K, et al. Simultaneous 68Ga-PSMA HBED-CC PET/MRI improves the localization of primary prostate cancer. Eur Urol 2016;70(5):829–36.

66. D'Amico AV, Whittington R, Malkowicz SB, et al. Biochemical outcome after radical prostatectomy, external beam radiation therapy, or interstitial radiation therapy for clinically localized prostate cancer. JAMA 1998;280(11):969–74.

67. Miller DC, Hafez KS, Stewart A, et al. Prostate carcinoma presentation, diagnosis, and staging. Cancer 2003;98(6):1169–78.

68. Maurer T, Gschwend JE, Rauscher I, et al. Diagnostic efficacy of (68)Gallium-PSMA positron emission tomography compared to conventional imaging for lymph node staging of 130 consecutive patients with intermediate to high risk prostate cancer. J Urol 2016;195(5):1436–43.

69. Cookson MS, Aus G, Burnett AL, et al. Variation in the definition of biochemical recurrence in patients treated for localized prostate cancer: the American Urological Association Prostate Guidelines for Localized Prostate Cancer Update Panel report and recommendations for a standard in the reporting of surgical outcomes. J Urol 2007;177(2):540–5.

70. Kwon O, Kim KB, Lee YI, et al. Salvage radiotherapy after radical prostatectomy: prediction of biochemical outcomes. PLoS One 2014;9(7):e103574.

71. Roehl KA, Han M, Ramos CG, et al. Cancer progression and survival rates following anatomical radical retropubic prostatectomy in 3,478 consecutive patients: long-term results. J Urol 2004;172(3): 910–4.

72. Afshar-Oromieh A, Haberkorn U, Schlemmer HP, et al. Comparison of PET/CT and PET/MRI hybrid systems using a 68Ga-labelled PSMA ligand for the diagnosis of recurrent prostate cancer: initial experience. Eur J Nucl Med Mol Imaging 2014;41(5):887–97.

73. Freitag MT, Radtke JP, Afshar-Oromieh A, et al. Local recurrence of prostate cancer after radical prostatectomy is at risk to be missed in 68Ga-PSMA-11-PET of PET/CT and PET/MRI: comparison with mpMRI integrated in simultaneous PET/MRI. Eur J Nucl Med Mol Imaging 2017;44(5):776–87.

74. Wright GL Jr, Grob BM, Haley C, et al. Upregulation of prostate-specific membrane antigen after androgen-deprivation therapy. Urology 1996;48(2): 326–34.

75. Baum RP, Kulkarni HR, Schuchardt C, et al. 177Lu-labeled prostate-specific membrane antigen radioligand therapy of metastatic castration-resistant prostate cancer: safety and efficacy. J Nucl Med 2016;57(7):1006–13.

76. Vallabhajosula S, Goldsmith SJ, Hamacher KA, et al. Prediction of myelotoxicity based on bone marrow radiation-absorbed dose: radioimmunotherapy studies using 90Y- and 177Lu-labeled J591 antibodies specific for prostate-specific membrane antigen. J Nucl Med 2005;46(5):850–8.

77. Hassan MM, Phan A, Li D, et al. Risk factors associated with neuroendocrine tumors: a U.S.-based case-control study. Int J Cancer 2008;123(4):867–73.

78. Frilling A, Sotiropoulos GC, Li J, et al. Multimodal management of neuroendocrine liver metastases. HPB (Oxford) 2010;12(6):361–79.

79. Strosberg J, El-Haddad G, Wolin E, et al. Phase 3 trial of 177Lu-Dotatate for Midgut neuroendocrine tumors. N Engl J Med 2017;376(2):125–35.

80. Yang J, Kan Y, Ge BH, et al. Diagnostic role of Gallium-68 DOTATOC and Gallium-68 DOTATATE PET in patients with neuroendocrine tumors: a meta-analysis. Acta Radiol 2014;55(4):389–98.

81. Buchmann I, Henze M, Engelbrecht S, et al. Comparison of 68Ga-DOTATOC PET and 111In-DTPAOC (Octreoscan) SPECT in patients with neuroendocrine tumours. Eur J Nucl Med Mol Imaging 2007; 34(10):1617–26.

82. Hope TA, Pampaloni MH, Flavell RR, et al. Somatostatin receptor PET/MRI for the evaluation of neuroendocrine tumors. Clin Transl Imaging 2017; 5:63.

83. Gaertner FC, Beer AJ, Souvatzoglou M, et al. Evaluation of feasibility and image quality of 68Ga-DOTA-TOC positron emission tomography/magnetic resonance in comparison with positron emission tomography/computed tomography in patients with neuroendocrine tumors. Invest Radiol 2013;48(5): 263–72.

84. Hope TA, Pampaloni MH, Nakakura E, et al. Simultaneous (68)Ga-DOTA-TOC PET/MRI with gadoxetate disodium in patients with neuroendocrine tumor. Abdom Imaging 2015;40(6):1432–40.

85. Sankowski AJ, Cwikla JB, Nowicki ML, et al. The clinical value of MRI using single-shot echoplanar DWI to identify liver involvement in patients with advanced gastroenteropancreatic-neuroendocrine tumors (GEP-NETs), compared to FSE T2 and FFE T1 weighted image after i.v. Gd-EOB-DTPA contrast enhancement. Med Sci Monit 2012;18(5):MT33–40.

86. Mayerhoefer ME, Ba-Ssalamah A, Weber M, et al. Gadoxetate-enhanced versus diffusion-weighted MRI for fused Ga-68-DOTANOC PET/MRI in patients with neuroendocrine tumours of the upper abdomen. Eur Radiol 2013;23(7):1978–85.

87. Giesel FL, Kratochwil C, Mehndiratta A, et al. Comparison of neuroendocrine tumor detection and characterization using DOTATOC-PET in correlation with contrast enhanced CT and delayed contrast enhanced MRI. Eur J Radiol 2012;81(10):2820–5.

88. Schreiter NF, Nogami M, Steffen I, et al. Evaluation of the potential of PET-MRI fusion for detection of liver metastases in patients with neuroendocrine tumours. Eur Radiol 2012;22(2):458–67.

89. Flechsig P, Zechmann CM, Schreiweis J, et al. Qualitative and quantitative image analysis of CT and MR imaging in patients with neuroendocrine liver metastases in comparison to (68)Ga-DOTATOC PET. Eur J Radiol 2015;84(8):1593–600.

90. Hofman MS, Lau WF, Hicks RJ. Somatostatin receptor imaging with 68Ga DOTATATE PET/CT: clinical utility, normal patterns, pearls, and pitfalls in interpretation. Radiographics 2015;35(2):500–16.

Printed and bound by CPI Group (UK) Ltd, Croydon, CR0 4YY

03/10/2024

01040383-0010